D1429698

Yoga Therapy

Yoga Therapy

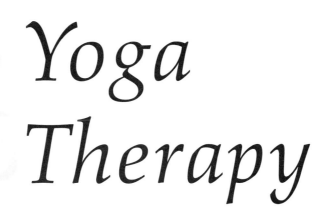

A Guide to the Therapeutic
Use of Yoga and Ayurveda for
Health and Fitness

A. G. MOHAN
AND INDRA MOHAN

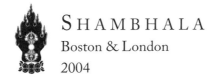

SHAMBHALA
Boston & London
2004

Shambhala Publications, Inc.
Horticultural Hall
300 Massachusetts Avenue
Boston, Massachusetts 02115
www.shambhala.com

© 2004 by A. G. Mohan and Indra Mohan

All rights reserved. No part of this book may be
reproduced in any form or by any means, electronic
or mechanical, including photocopying, recording,
or by any information storage and retrieval system,
without permission in writing from the publisher.

9 8 7 6 5 4 3 2

Printed in the United States of America

♾ This edition is printed on acid-free paper that meets the
American National Standards Institute Z39.48 Standard.
Distributed in the United States by Random House, Inc.,
and in Canada by Random House of Canada Ltd

Library of Congress Cataloging-in-Publication Data
Mohan, A. G. (Angarai Ganesha). 1945–
Yoga therapy: a guide to the therapeutic use of yoga and
ayurveda for health and fitness/A. G. Mohan and Indra
Mohan.—1st ed.
p. cm.
ISBN 1-59030-131-5 (pbk.: alk. paper)
1. Yoga—Health apsects. 2. Medicine, Ayurvedic. I. Mohan,
Indra. II. Title.
RA781.7.M643 2004
613.7'046—dc22
2004013758

Contents

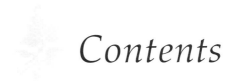

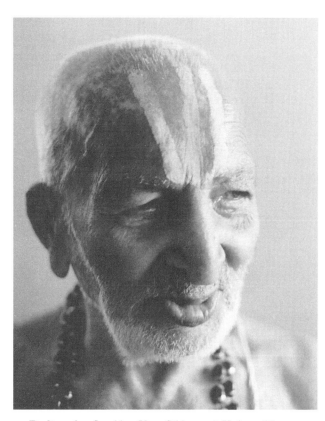

Dedicated to Samkhya Yoga Sikhamani, Vedanta Vageesa,
Veda Kesari, Nyayacharya Mimamsa Tirtha, Mimamsa Ratna,
Yogacharya Shri T. Krishnamacharya

Preface

My wife, Indra, and I have been teaching yoga for over twenty-five years. Since the demise of my teacher Sri T. Krishnamacharya in 1989, we have been studying Ayurveda and other fields related to physical and mental health in great detail. Our son, Ganesh, has been practicing yoga since childhood. After studying Ayurveda in college for four years, he is currently studying Western medicine and is now in his final year of school. A few years ago, he suggested that we present the practice of yoga in a systematic, logical manner. Our daughter, Nitya, who has also been practicing yoga since childhood, is herself a yoga teacher, and she agreed to help. This book is a family endeavor. We have tried to make this book clear, rational, and unambiguous. Wherever possible, we have explained not only what should be done but also why it should be done that way.

The main portion of this book deals with the practice of asana and pranayama. However, we have also explained the fundamental approach of Ayurveda and how it can complement yoga in providing a comprehensive health system. The practical application of these principles is illustrated by numerous case studies of people we have treated over the last three decades. We have also touched upon some other important topics, including the relationship between asanas and the *dosha*s, the approach to using pranayama in yoga therapy, the concepts of *brmhana* and *langhana*, as well as the principles of Ayurvedic diet. As a result, this book contains material for both yoga practitioners and yoga teachers.

Special thanks to Beth Frankl, Associate Editor, Shambhala Publications, Inc., for her valuable suggestions and editorial assistance.

PART ONE

Yoga for Fitness

An Introduction to Yoga and Ayurveda 1

Y OGA AND A YURVEDA form a comprehensive and integrated working model to address all aspects of our health and well-being—both for maintaining health and for resolving conditions of ill health. On the basis of this model, it is possible to explain how six factors—diet, environment, lifestyle, exercise (in the form of asana), breathing techniques (in the form of pranayama), and mental techniques—can be used to restore balance to both body and mind.

YOGA AND AYURVEDA: BODY AND MIND

Yoga deals primarily with the management of our mind. It explains in great detail how we can increase our mental balance and clarity.

The cornerstone of the approach of yoga is the model of the three *guna*s.

Ayurveda is mainly concerned with how to maintain and restore balance in the qualities and functions in our body. For this, it uses the model of the five elements and the model of the three *dosha*s. It explains how food and environment affect the qualities and functions in our body on the basis of these two models.

Although yoga does not explain the effect of food and environment on the body and mind in detail, it does suggest broad guidelines for a healthy diet and lifestyle, based on the same model that Ayurveda uses.

Similarly, Ayurveda focuses on healing the body, but it also deals with the treatment of psychological disorders using the same model of the three gunas that yoga does.

The approach taken in this book draws on the knowledge contained within several ancient texts, especially the *Yoga-Sutras* of Patanjali and the *Caraka-Samhita*.

THE QUALITIES AND FUNCTIONS OF OBJECTS

All objects have certain qualities and certain functions. Consider a pink rose, for example. It has color—pink, in this case—and a certain shape. It is soft to touch and fragile. It has a characteristic fragrance. All these are qualities of the rose. On the stalk of the rose is a thorn. It is green or brown in color. It has a pointed shape. It is hard and sharp to the touch. These are qualities of the thorn. An apple is firm to touch but not as hard as the thorn. It too has a characteristic smell. Unlike the rose and the thorn, it is sweet in taste. All of these are qualities of the apple.

All objects in this world, including our body and mind, have some qualities and some functions. No object exists without any qualities at all.

Just as objects do not exist without any qualities at all, qualities do not exist separate from objects. For example, the color green does not exist separate from an object. We see the color green, but it is always present only on the basis of some object: a green leaf, a green apple, or a green door, for example. Never do we see "a green." We always see "a green something."

Therefore, the connection between an object and the qualities it possesses is insepa-

rable, and consequently, an object is defined by the qualities it possesses. That is why we usually describe an object by stating its qualities—the qualities of an object are usually the adjectives we use to describe it. For example, a pink rose is one that has the color pink as its quality. A sweet apple is one that has the quality of tasting sweet. Similarly, adjectives like *green*, *brown*, *hard*, *firm*, and *soft* are all qualities of the object being described.

The qualities of one particular object make that object what it is. Among these qualities, those that are specific to a particular object make that object different from other similar objects. A paper rose, for instance, may be similar to a real one in color and shape, but it does not have the same velvet texture or pleasant fragrance. Among real roses, a yellow rose differs from a pink rose in its color. Even between two roses of the same color there are small differences in shape. It is the differences in the qualities of objects that allow us to distinguish one object from another.

Between the qualities and the functions an object possesses, the qualities are of greater importance to us, because they usually determine the object's function. For example, an eraser is soft and compressible and can peel away when rubbed on a surface. It is these qualities in the eraser that endow it with the function of removing pencil marks when it is rubbed against them. An eraser cannot be made of steel. Steel is hard. If we rub a piece of steel on a paper that has pencil marks on it, the steel will not erase the pencil marks. Instead, it will tear the paper. Hardness is a quality of steel that confers on it the function of eroding or breaking substances with which it comes in contact.

Because the qualities of an object largely determine its functions, we must know the qualities of an object in order to judge the effect it can have on our body and mind.

HEALTH IS A BALANCE

The various structures and systems in our body have many different qualities and functions. Health is a balance between extremes in the qualities and functions of our body. For example, our skin has a layer of lipids (oils) on it. This natural level of oiliness is necessary to resist infections and maintain the integrity of the skin. Excessively dry skin is undesirable. The other extreme—excessively oily skin—is also undesirable. Therefore, lipids, or the quality of being oily, must be expressed within certain limits in skin if it is to be healthy. Either excess or deficiency can lead to ill health. Similarly, consider the heart's function of rhythmic contraction. This must occur without excessive force or increase in rate, nor with decreased force or rate. To maintain health, the functioning of any body part or system must fall within a certain range of intensity.

THE BODY AND THE ENVIRONMENT

As we know, various qualities and functions exist in our body and in the inanimate and animate things in our environment. We are in constant contact with the environment. Our body and the environment have several similar qualities, and opposite ones as well. On the basis of this similarity or dissimilarity in qualities, our interaction with the environment inevitably changes the qualities in our body. The nature of the changes is determined by the specific qualities of the objects and the type and duration of our connection with them.

For example, heat is present in the environment and in our body. Hot surroundings can, obviously, increase the heat in our body. This is a simple physical phenomenon. But our body is a biological system in dynamic equilibrium. Changing any of our body's qualities will result in changes in various other qualities and functions. For example, in response to increased heat, there will be an increase in perspiration.

Our body is constantly subject to change because of its interactions with the environment outside. The cornerstone of the approach of Ayurveda to restoring or maintaining health and balance is this: We can intelligently change the qualities and functions of our body by controlling our interactions with our environment and by altering the food we eat.

Food is the most important factor in our environment that affects our body's function. Not only does the environment around us influence us from outside, it becomes part of our body every day in the form of the food we eat. Food is therefore a potent modifier of body qualities and functions.

Further, by means of changes in body movement, by the use of breathing techniques, and by directly or indirectly changing our thought processes, we can influence the qualities and functions of our body and mind to restore or to maintain balance. Yoga explains how we can do this.

Let us begin with the qualities of the outside environment.

THE FIVE FORMS OF MATTER

What qualities can an object possess? If we touch a piece of wood, we may find it hard. But a piece of velvet will be soft to the touch. If we try to lift a large box of metal tools, we may find it heavy, but the same box filled with cotton balls will seem light. We may touch a surface and say it is dry or oily or maybe wet. Obviously, the list is endless.

We cannot work effectively with innumerable qualities. We need to classify or group the important qualities into a limited number of broad categories. This categorization must have some logical basis and must also be of some use in maintaining and restoring health. These qualities can be placed in five groups: the five forms of matter. A simple and easily observable classification that both yoga and Ayurveda adopt is the five forms of matter (sometimes called the five elements): earth, water, fire, air, and space. Each of these five entities is a physical constituent of our world. Each has several qualities and functions. Together, they span a wide range of qualities, from heat to cold, dry to wet, light to heavy, hard to soft, and so on.

As we discuss this further, you will see that this is a rather simplistic classification, but one that is easily comprehensible and verifiable by direct observation.

In this classification, the words do not refer to the actual physical entities of earth, water, fire, air, or space that we see around us. They are not physical substances at all. They are simply names for a group of qualities and their associated functions.

We use these five categories—earth, water, fire, air, and space—because the groups of qualities we find in these entities are seen together in many other objects as well. The physical entities themselves are merely the most well-known, universally present examples of these qualities occurring together.

By *earth*, for example, we do not refer to sand or rock but only the qualities, such as hardness, dryness, stability, and heaviness, that are found in it. These qualities are commonly found together in many objects, but the classic example among such objects is the earth itself. Similarly, *water* refers to qualities such as wetness, coldness, liquidity, and the tendency to adhere and bind. These qualities also commonly occur together in many objects, but the classic example is water itself. In the same way, air is the most easily observable example of such qualities as movement, lightness, and dryness occurring together in one object, though any other gas would share similar qualities.

In other words, the basis of the theory is not that there are five elements or forms of matter that make up the world, each having the listed qualities. Rather, the world has myriad qualities and functions that we group under these five categories for convenience. We name these categories after the most common examples of objects in which these qualities are combined.

For example, consider this statement: Oil has a predominance of the water element. Oil, as we know, does not mix with water at all. Oil most certainly does not contain water. So, what does this statement mean? It means only that oil has some of the qualities listed under the heading of the water element. These include the tendency to bind or stick and the quality of liquidity.

To give another example, bones are predominantly composed of the earth element. Earth, or sand, is mainly silicon dioxide. Bones have a matrix mostly of calcium compounds. Although there is no earth in our bones, our bones are hard and strong and a little rough. These are all qualities that we group under the earth element. Therefore, we can say that bones contain the earth element.

THE THREE DOSHAS

Our body is a living entity. It is a complex biological system, not merely a physical object. Therefore, the simple classification of the five forms of matter is insufficient to work with the complexities of body function. To work with the qualities and functions of our body, we have to group them in a manner that takes into account the way in which they are related within the body, and not the way they are related in the world outside.

To address this, Ayurveda groups body qualities and functions under a different classification. It suggests three groups, called the three doshas in Sanskrit. The three doshas in Ayurveda are a grouping of body qualities and functions that takes into account their interactions in the body. Both in maintaining health and in the treatment of illnesses, Ayurveda uses this classification as a working basis.

The three doshas are known as Vata, Pitta, and Kapha. Broadly, they relate to the classification of the five elements as follows: The

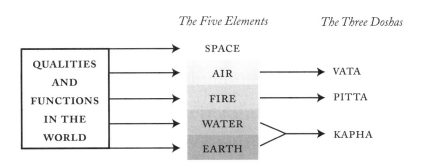

Fig. 1.1. The relation between the five elements and the three doshas.

qualities attributed to air are linked to Vata in the body. Under Pitta come the qualities of fire, and under Kapha are grouped the qualities of water and earth. Space is common to all three doshas (fig. 1.1).

The key body qualities under Vata are dryness, lightness, and some degree of coldness. The main function under Vata is movement of all types, including that involved in breathing.

The key body quality under Pitta is heat. Heat in the body is a product of metabolic activity, and so the various metabolic activities in the body are included under Pitta.

Kapha, the third dosha, comprises qualities like coldness, stability, and the ability to bind or hold structures together. Functions associated with maintaining the structural integrity of body parts are included under Kapha.

In practice, it is useful to limit the important qualities to a manageable number. Ayurveda suggests twenty easily observable qualities. We can define or describe several others, but most can be placed under one of these twenty qualities, or under a combination of two or more of these twenty (fig. 1.2).

Similar and Opposing Qualities

These twenty important qualities are distributed among the three doshas. In this grouping, some qualities are present under more than one dosha. But the doshas also have some opposing qualities. That is, there are areas of similarity and opposition among the three doshas. This results in considerable

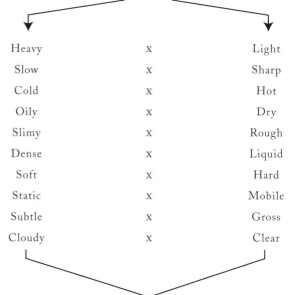

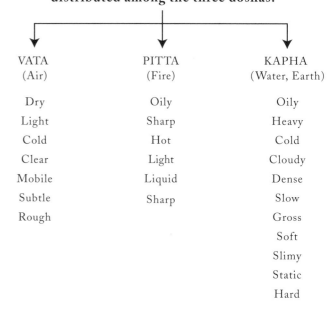

Fig. 1.2. The distribution of important qualities among the three doshas.

complexity but also in a greater approximation of reality, because the qualities in our body systems interact in several supportive and opposing ways, as in our classification among the doshas.

For example, Vata and Pitta share the quality of lightness, and the opposite quality—heaviness—belongs to Kapha. Pitta is the only dosha with the quality of heat—the other two doshas have coldness as a quality (more in Kapha than in Vata). Similarly, dryness is present in Vata, and the opposite quality of wetness or oiliness is found in both Pitta and Kapha, though more in the latter (fig. 1.3).

An Imbalance of Doshas

Just as the five forms of matter are not the physical entities in the external world that bear their names, the three doshas are not substances in the body. They are a grouping of qualities and associated functions.

An important purpose of this classification is to help in logically grouping imbalances in body function, so that restoring balance is made easier. That is why Ayurveda describes various physical illnesses in terms of imbalances in the doshas—for example, as an increase in Vata or an increase in Pitta.

When we speak of one of the doshas being out of balance—as being increased or decreased—it means that one or more of its qualities and functions is out of balance; that is, those particular qualities or functions are being expressed excessively or are deficient. Therefore, a simple statement like "Vata is increased" is not a complete description of an imbalance in the body, because it does not explain what qualities or functions of Vata are increased or where in the body this imbalance has occurred. Similarly, it gives us an idea of what the general therapeutic approach could be, but it does not tell us the specific therapy we should follow.

For example, a decrease in the structural integrity of the cartilage within a joint is seen in osteoarthritis. The quality of binding and

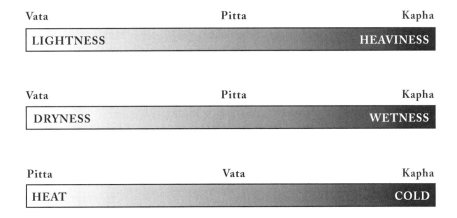

Fig. 1.3. The relation between the three pairs of important qualities and the three doshas.

maintaining structural integrity belongs to Kapha. The opposite quality—dryness and a loss of structural integrity—belongs to Vata. Therefore, osteoarthritis is a condition in which the quality of dryness, belonging to Vata, is increased in the joints. Generic measures can be suggested to address this imbalance (the increase in Vata), but to accurately tailor therapeutic measures to the problem, it is important to identify the specific qualities and functions that are out of balance, as well as the affected site or tissue.

THE THREE GUNAS

The approach of the three gunas underlies all major systems of Vedic philosophy, including yoga. A clear understanding of this approach is essential to comprehending the psychology of yoga—the reasoning behind the various practices suggested in the *Yoga-Sutras* of Patanjali (the most comprehensive and authoritative exposition of yoga) and the content of several Upanishads. This approach is also used by Ayurveda to work with disorders of mental balance, both of thoughts and emotions.

As we have seen, objects in the world, including our own bodies, have various qualities and functions. The mind has no form, color, touch, taste, sound, or smell. In other words, the mind is not an object that can be perceived by the senses. In our experience, our mind consists of various thoughts and emotions. Emotions may be strong enough to be clearly obvious to us. For example, an emotion like intense anger, which we have all experienced, forces itself into our field of attention. At other times, the same emotions may be present in a more subtle and complex fashion, making it difficult for us to identify the nature of the emotion or its cause. The thoughts in our mind are usually associated with or prompted by this underlying complex jumble of changing emotions. The complexities of our thoughts and emotions have been analyzed in terms of the three gunas.

The three gunas are *sattva*, *rajas*, and *tamas*. We say that our mind is in a state of sattva when we experience contentment, quiet, and clarity. We have all experienced this to varying degrees, usually when we attain something that we desire greatly or in places of great natural beauty. Sattva is not exultation but the feeling of contentment and completeness that stems from a tranquil mind. The less we experience fluctuation in the mind, the greater the depth of completeness and contentment we feel. Sattva is a state of mind that arises because of a decrease in the mental fluctuations caused by desire—either temporarily by the fulfillment of a particular desire or more permanently through the means suggested by yoga.

Rajas is a state of mind in which we are driven to action by desire or dislike. Contact with some object, person, or situation, or simply the memory of it in our mind, evokes feelings of desire or dislike. On this basis, we act either to attain or to avoid that object, person, or situation. This state of compulsive or driven activity is the state of rajas. We do not have a choice in this, because we will be unhappy if we do not act. If we have the necessary skills and knowledge, and if the circumstances are favorable, we will be successful in attaining what we desire or in avoiding or removing what we dislike. Then our mind will return to the earlier state of greater contentment and completeness. In other words, the sattva in our mind increases when the fluctuation due to desire or dislike (rajas) is decreased to its former level.

But we do not always have the knowledge and ability required to do this, and circumstances are not always favorable to us. Therefore, we may face a situation in which we are not clear about what to do to satisfy our desire or reduce our unhappiness. This state of mind in which we lack clarity is a state of tamas. When our mind is not clear, we may not act when we should, or we may act when we should not. Thus, tamas can manifest as inactivity or retarded activity. However, if the drive to do something is too strong—that is, if the rajas in our mind is high as well—we may act blindly, without clarity about what should be done.

Sattva Is Our Natural State

Sattva is the state of mind that all of us want to be in—complete and fulfilled. Yoga and Ayurveda suggest that this is our natural state of mind, and rajas and tamas represent aberrations, deviations from this natural state. To understand why, let us look a little further into how the outcome of our actions and therefore their success or failure is affected by the state of mind from which we do those actions.

When sattva is dominant in our mind, we act with awareness and calmness, undisturbed by the possible failure or success of the action. Our mental balance is not dependent on the outcome of the action because we do not bind our happiness and contentment to our success. This allows us to act or not act with equal ease. That is, we not only have the ability to act with calm efficiency, but we are also free from the compulsion to act: We can withdraw with no misgivings if that is what needs to be done. When we act from a state of sattva, we can do what is required—no more and no less—and never lose our mental calm.

When rajas dominates our mind, we may act with awareness and clarity, but always with vigor and compulsion, and our mind will be colored by expectation and anxiety regarding the outcome of the action. Our happiness is bound to the outcome. We feel that we will be happier—more content—if the outcome is successful. That is, the action is driven by the underlying feeling of discontent. The anxiety, expectation, and drive to act affect our mental calm and hamper our ability to act with balance.

When tamas dominates our mind, there is lack of clarity about what should or should not be done. This results in inaction or inappropriate action.

To further our mental health and balance, to know what will bring us and others happiness, and to act on this knowledge with maximum clarity, we need to develop a sattvic state of mind in preference to rajasic or tamasic states.

The interaction of the qualities and

functions of our body with the physical world, such as food and other objects in our environment, is much more predictable than the interaction of objects, persons, or situations with our mind. The same object, person, or situation may induce different states of mind in different people depending on their relationship to it. That is why the same object can be a cause of happiness to one person and unhappiness to another.

For example, a person may inspire feelings of love, trust, and satisfaction (sattva) in his or her partner. The same person may be a source of infatuation and blind desire (tamas) to a stalker. An enemy may view the person as an obstacle to be removed—a cause for anger (rajas).

The Three Gunas Are Constantly Changing

We are always alternating between contentment and desire, clarity and confusion. Our state of mind is altered by time and by the object we are thinking about. We may have one state of mind at a particular time in relation to an object or person, but our relationship to the same object or person may change over time so that it later induces in us a different state of mind.

Therefore, the gunas are not absolutes that pervade our mind. Rather, our mind constantly shifts among the states of mind represented by the gunas, in varying intensities. In other words, we can say that all three gunas are always present in our mind, but, at any

moment, one will be stronger than the others, only to be overshadowed by the ascent of another in a short while.

From this constant fluctuation and rotation among gunas in our mind, it naturally follows that though some of us may have a predominance of one of the gunas, they are not fixed character traits. That is, we all have all three of these states of mind to varying degrees. This means that a normally rajas-dominated person may respond in a tamasic manner in some situations or at some times. Yoga and Ayurveda suggest that lasting changes in our state of mind that will lead to greater contentment (sattva) can be brought about by sustained effort—which would be fundamentally impossible if the gunas were fixed character traits.

The gunas are also affected by our diet. Proper nutrition is essential to maintain a clear mind. However, the connection between the qualities in the mind and the food that we eat is a complex subject that requires much explanation and is beyond the scope of this book.

Increasing Sattva, Decreasing Rajas and Tamas

We can always relate to objects so that the balance of our mind is not disturbed. Balance and clarity are a state of our mind—they do not arise from the objects we come in contact with; they arise because of our mind's response to such contact. To be in a state of sattva is to instill in our mind such deep and unshakable steadiness that our balance, contentment, and clarity are not compromised by our interactions with objects, people, and situations. To do this, rajas and tamas need to be decreased, as they indicate a descent into imbalance and a lack of clarity.

Yoga deals in great detail with the means to increase sattva and reduce rajas and tamas so that we can move from our present state of fluctuating contentment to a state of greater quietness and tranquillity. Ayurveda adopts the same basic approach but places more emphasis on the therapy of mental illnesses—to move from mental illness to normality.

Principles of Movement and Breathing

2

IF YOU OPEN any book on yoga, you are likely to find drawings or photos of people in various body positions. These body positions have names, traditionally given in Sanskrit. Most of these names end with the word *asana*. Essentially, asanas are movements of the body or stays in specific body positions, practiced with appropriate breathing. Why should we practice asanas? What can they do for us? Asanas are, at the very least, a form of exercise, and we must expect from them the benefits that we would from other forms of exercise. Ideally, an exercise program should lead us toward greater physical and mental health. In other words, it should help promote the following:

- Strength
- Flexibility
- Structural alignment
- Proper functioning of various body systems
- Mental steadiness

We require all five for good health, and asanas can give us all five if they are done correctly. Further, asanas can help heal various imbalances in our body and mind. This chapter explains what constitutes asanas, and the important principles of how movement and breathing should be done in asanas so that you derive all their benefits. Chapters 3, 4, and 5 explain an equally important process: how to tailor your asana practice to suit your physical and mental makeup and your particular needs.

WHAT IS AN ASANA?

In yoga texts, the word *asana* is used to refer to any position of the body. Though the name of any asana refers only to that specific body position, the process of doing that asana involves moving into and out of that position as well. Therefore, when we speak of an asana, the following three steps are implied (fig. 2.1):

1. Movement into the asana from a prior body position
2. Staying in the asana
3. Movement out of the asana, usually back to the body position we started from

Each of these steps should be done with appropriate breathing. Therefore, an asana involves a controlled movement of the body and a stay in a certain body position, and it is done with specific, regulated breathing. We will discuss each of these components further.

Performing any asana simply involves movement into, staying in, and movement out of the asana, with the appropriate breathing. In one sense, each asana is just a name for a certain body position. It is not very different from a word like *squatting*—a word that serves to indicate a certain position of the body.

It is not the case that the position of the asana, undertaken with mathematical preci-

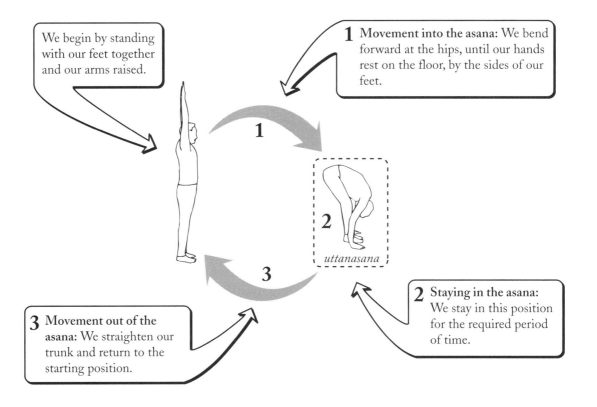

We begin by standing with our feet together and our arms raised.

1 **Movement into the asana:** We bend forward at the hips, until our hands rest on the floor, by the sides of our feet.

uttanasana

2 **Staying in the asana:** We stay in this position for the required period of time.

3 **Movement out of the asana:** We straighten our trunk and return to the starting position.

Fig. 2.1. The three steps in doing *uttanasana*.

sion, results in occult benefits. Asanas do not have intrinsic benefits distinct from those that result from the movements and breathing. The effect of an asana is simply the effect of the movement of the body and the flow of the breath. Similar movement and breathing will, quite naturally, have similar effects. For example, logically speaking, squatting with our feet together (*utkatasana*) will have largely the same effect as squatting with our feet a few inches apart. Similarly, bending forward halfway at the hips to rest our arms on a chair will have an effect similar to bending forward to touch our toes (*uttanasana*), only the effect will be less intense.

Our goal should not be to place our body in the position of an asana. Rather, we must seek to develop the strength and flexibility that will enable us to assume such a position. That is, the goal should not be the asana itself but the attributes of the physical fitness that are implied in the ability to assume that body position. This is a crucial distinction, for it is possible to assume some asanas without developing such fitness. To focus on achieving the ideal form of an asana without paying adequate attention to the effect of the practice on the structural qualities of the body is to lose sight of the true goal of asana practice.

MOVEMENT IN ASANAS

When we do an asana, we move from one body position to another, stay in the second body position for some time, and then move out of it, usually back to the first body position. The following three factors determine the nature of any asana:

1. The body position that we start from
2. The parts of our body that we move
3. The direction in which we move them

The body position we stay in—that is, the body position that we call the asana—is a consequence of the initial body position and the nature of the movement we make. That is, the starting body position and the type of movement we make will naturally determine what final body position we reach.

Each of these three factors can be divided into four types. Therefore, in asanas, we use four starting body positions, four parts of the body, and four directions of movement. All asanas can be derived by combining these factors in various ways. The traditional asanas are body positions derived from a specific combination of these components. Their value is not that they are traditional but that they are particularly useful in developing and maintaining health.

The four types of starting body positions are standing, seated, lying, and inverted (fig. 2.2). Standing, seated, and lying positions are common body positions that we are used to being in throughout our daily activities. In asanas we make movements in the inverted position as well. This position is unfamiliar to us and must therefore be used only after adequate preparation. All other starting body positions are modifications or derivations of these four basic ones.

The four parts of the body that we move in asanas are the arms, legs, head, and trunk (fig. 2.3). The four important directions of movement are forward, backward, twisting, and lateral (fig. 2.4). In figure 2.5 you can see a summary of the components of movement and breathing and how they constitute asanas.

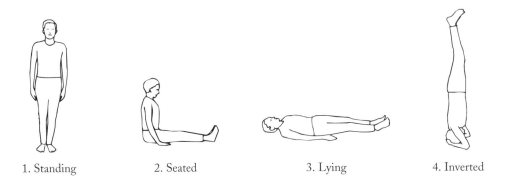

1. Standing   2. Seated   3. Lying   4. Inverted

Fig. 2.2. The four groups of starting body positions used in asanas.

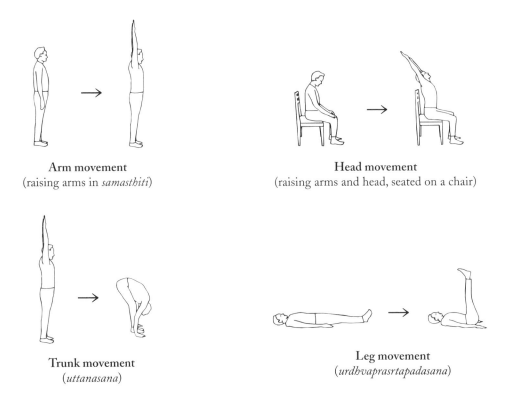

Arm movement
(raising arms in *samasthiti*)

Head movement
(raising arms and head, seated on a chair)

Trunk movement
(*uttanasana*)

Leg movement
(*urdhvaprasrtapadasana*)

Fig. 2.3. The four body parts that are moved in asanas.

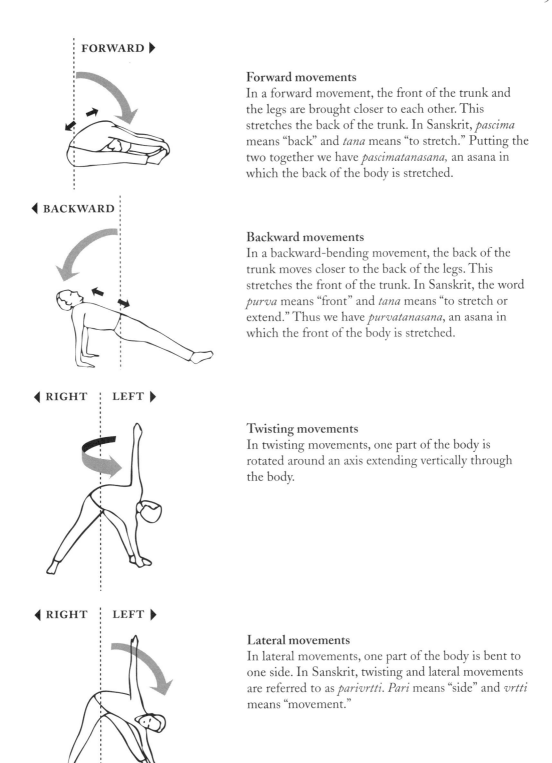

Forward movements

In a forward movement, the front of the trunk and the legs are brought closer to each other. This stretches the back of the trunk. In Sanskrit, *pascima* means "back" and *tana* means "to stretch." Putting the two together we have *pascimatanasana*, an asana in which the back of the body is stretched.

Backward movements

In a backward-bending movement, the back of the trunk moves closer to the back of the legs. This stretches the front of the trunk. In Sanskrit, the word *purva* means "front" and *tana* means "to stretch or extend." Thus we have *purvatanasana*, an asana in which the front of the body is stretched.

Twisting movements

In twisting movements, one part of the body is rotated around an axis extending vertically through the body.

Lateral movements

In lateral movements, one part of the body is bent to one side. In Sanskrit, twisting and lateral movements are referred to as *parivrtti. Pari* means "side" and *vrtti* means "movement."

Fig. 2.4. The four directions of movements in asanas.

Four components of the breathing cycle	Four body positions	Four parts of the body being moved	Four directions of movement
1. Inhalation	1. Standing	1. Arms	1. Forward
2. Holding	2. Seated	2. Legs	2. Backward
3. Exhalation	3. Lying	3. Head	3. Twisting
4. Suspension	4. Inverted	4. Trunk	4. Lateral

BREATHING   AND   **MOVEMENT**

TOGETHER CONSTITUTE

ALL ASANAS

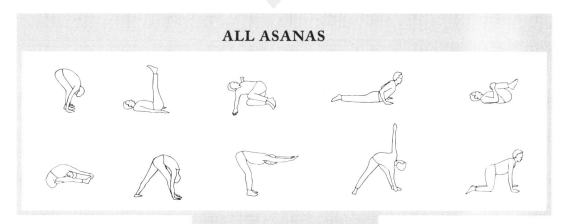

WHICH, WHEN DONE PROPERLY, CAN PROMOTE

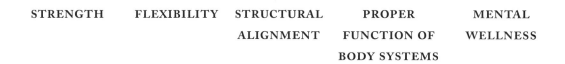

STRENGTH   FLEXIBILITY   STRUCTURAL ALIGNMENT   PROPER FUNCTION OF BODY SYSTEMS   MENTAL WELLNESS

Fig. 2.5. Asanas consist of breathing and movement, each having several components. When these components are combined and practiced properly, they can provide benefits in all aspects of our health.

There are two important features of movement in asanas:

- Asanas include movements in all three axes.
- Asanas may involve more than one movement, done simultaneously or sequentially.

Movements in All Three Axes

We live in a world that has three physical dimensions. All movements of the body take place in one or more of these three planes or dimensions. We have already classified movement in asanas into four types: forward-bending, backward-bending, twisting, and lateral movements. Forward and backward movements take place in the sagittal plane but are opposite in direction. Twisting is a movement in the transverse plane. Lateral bending is a movement in the lateral or coronal plane.

In the course of our daily activities, we move repeatedly in only some directions, and the range of our movement is limited. For example, we rarely do full twisting movements. Lateral-bending movements are even more uncommon in our normal activities. In asanas, we can include movements in all three planes—that is, in all possible directions—and with the full range of movement. This is very important for retaining the ability to do full and free movements, especially as we age.

More Than One Movement

We usually do more than one movement in each asana, either simultaneously or in

sequence. Even simple asanas commonly involve more than one movement. The net effect of an asana is the result of the interaction of the effects of the component movements. The first example (fig. 2.6) shows how the component movements in one asana can be opposing in nature, while the second example shows how they can support each other. (The examples may be clearer if you come back to them at the end of this chapter, after reading the discussion about the connection between breathing and movement in asanas and their effects on the spine.)

The important practical point is that the effect of an asana can be changed by varying the component movements. For example, in *uttanasana*, as you bend down, instead of keeping your arms stretched out, you can sweep your arms backward to rest them on your lower back. This will round your upper back more than if you keep your arms stretched out, and it will also rest your shoulders. You may choose to do *uttanasana* in this manner if you are doing it to relieve the stress created by a strenuous backward-bending movement, or after an asana in which the shoulders and arms have been placed under strain.

The science in asanas lies in understanding the effects of the component movements in an asana, their interactions, and their relationship to the breathing process and the spine. The art in asana practice is in assessing yourself and making it relevant to your needs and respectful of your individuality. In chapter 5 we discuss the broad categories of changes that can be

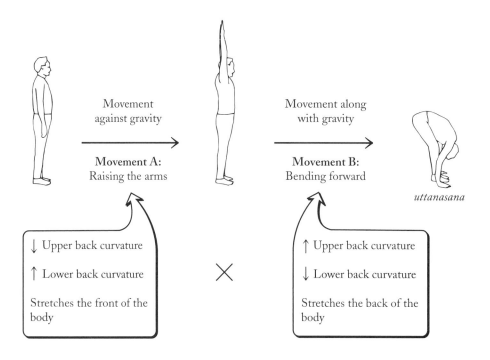

Fig. 2.6. Two opposing movements in one asana: raising the arms and bending forward in *uttanasana*.

made to the individual movements in asanas and their common uses.

Example 1: Two movements with differing effects in one asana. Classically, in practically all asanas done from the standing position, the arms are raised before the movement into the asana. This is an example of two movements with differing effects occurring in sequence in one asana.

For instance, when we do *uttanasana*, we first raise our arms, and then we bend forward from the hips (fig. 2.6). The forward-bending movement stretches our hamstrings and helps to increase hip flexibility. It also stretches our

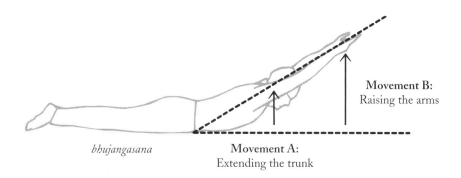

Fig. 2.7. Two supporting movements in one asana: extending the trunk and raising the arms in *bhujangasana*.

back, decreasing the curvature of our lower back and increasing the curvature of our upper back. It is a movement that goes along with gravity and mostly increases flexibility rather than strength.

Raising our arms before we bend down has an opposite effect on the back. It decreases the curvature of our upper back and increases the curvature of our lower back. It also opens out the front of our body, unlike the forward-bending movement that follows. That is, raising the arms resembles a backward-bending movement in its effect, while the movement into *uttanasana* is a forward-bending movement. The net effect of *uttanasana* is the result of the interaction of these two component movements, with their differing characteristics.

Example 2: Two movements with supporting effects in one asana. In many backward-bending asanas like *bhujangasana,* we raise our arms as we extend or arch our trunk (fig. 2.7). The two movements—arm raising and back extension—are done simultaneously. Since raising our arms is similar to a backward-bending movement, it supports the main backward-bending movement, resulting in increased extension of the back.

Example 3: A sequence of several movements. In the practice of asanas, sequences of more than two or three movements, as shown in figure 2.8, are not uncommon. Usually, adjacent movements in such sequences are opposite in nature, like a gentle backward bend following a forward bend. The reason for such an arrangement is discussed in chapter 4.

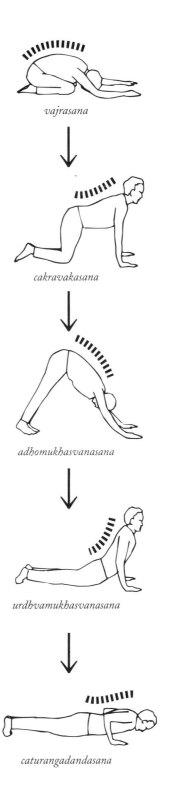

vajrasana

cakravakasana

adhomukhasvanasana

urdhvamukhasvanasana

caturangadandasana

Fig. 2.8. A sequence of five asanas, with opposite flexion-extension movements in consecutive asanas.

BREATHING IN ASANAS

Inhalation and Exhalation

Inhalation is the active process of drawing air into the lungs. It is an active process driven by muscular contraction. The muscles that make inhalation possible are the diaphragm and the intercostal muscles. When we inhale, the diaphragm descends, and the intercostal muscles move the ribs and sternum upward and forward. Both of these increase the volume of the chest and decrease the pressure within the lungs. When the pressure within our lungs falls below atmospheric pressure, air flows into our lungs from outside.

Inhalation opens out the front of our body. The contraction of the intercostal muscles makes the chest expand. The downward movement of the diaphragm compresses the contents of our abdomen and pushes the front wall of our abdomen outward. Therefore, both the chest and abdomen are expanded or opened out by inhalation.

Exhalation is the process of expelling air from the lungs. Normal unconscious exhalation is a passive process. When the muscles responsible for inhalation relax, the elastic recoil of our lungs expels the air within them. Muscle contraction is not required for normal unconscious exhalation. But when we consciously deepen or extend exhalation, our abdominal muscles are contracted. Contraction of the abdominal muscles compresses the contents of the abdomen and pushes the diaphragm upward. When the diaphragm moves upward, it compresses the lungs and expels the air from them more completely.

Exhalation tends to collapse the front of the body. It is associated with the inward movement of the chest and abdomen. This effect is increased when we consciously extend and deepen exhalation, as we do in asana practice. Pausing after inhalation or exhalation extends its effect. We can inhale or exhale for only a limited length of time. If we wish to further prolong the effect of inhalation, we can hold our breath for a few seconds after inhalation. Similarly, to prolong the effect of exhalation, we can suspend breathing for a few seconds after exhalation. In short, holding our breath after inhalation is like extending inhalation. Suspending breathing after exhalation is like extending exhalation. We use both in the practice of asanas.

Figure 2.9 summarizes the characteristics of these four components of the breathing cycle.

The Connection between Breathing and Movement

We breathe continuously throughout our lives. Expansion and relaxation of the chest and abdomen are integral to the process of breathing. Movements in asanas also open out or compress the chest and abdomen as we breathe in and out. Therefore, both breathing and movement affect, and are affected by, the shape of the body. Consequently, they are inextricably and naturally linked.

We must use this connection intelligently in the practice of asanas. When we move in

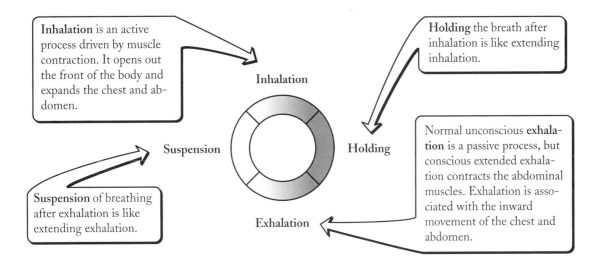

Inhalation is an active process driven by muscle contraction. It opens out the front of the body and expands the chest and abdomen.

Holding the breath after inhalation is like extending inhalation.

Suspension of breathing after exhalation is like extending exhalation.

Normal unconscious **exhalation** is a passive process, but conscious extended exhalation contracts the abdominal muscles. Exhalation is associated with the inward movement of the chest and abdomen.

Inhalation

Suspension

Holding

Exhalation

Fig. 2.9. Characteristics of the four components of the breathing cycle.

asanas, if we simultaneously use the correct component of the breathing cycle, our breathing will support the movement and increase its effect. If we combine movement with an opposing component of the breathing cycle, our breathing will hinder the movement or be hindered by it. Combining movement and breathing inappropriately will create conflict in the body and can adversely affect our health.

Four Rules for Combining Movement and Breathing

1. Do movements that open out the front of the body on inhalation. Backward-bending movements stretch the front of the body. So does raising the arms or the head. As we have seen, inhalation has a similar effect—it also opens out the front of the body. Therefore, backward-bending movements, raising the

arms, and raising the head should all be done on inhalation.

2. Do movements that compress the front of the body on exhalation. Forward-bending movements stretch the back of the body and compress the front of the body. As we saw, exhalation has a similar effect—it collapses or contracts the front of the body. Therefore, forward-bending movements should be done on exhalation.

Try inhaling while twisting or bending your trunk to one side. You will find that you cannot breathe in fully. This is because twisting and lateral-bending movements restrict the expansion of your chest and abdomen. Therefore, these movements should also be done on exhalation. That is, forward-bending, twisting, and lateral movements should all be done on exhalation.

These movements must not be done on inhalation. If you do these movements on inhalation, you will be compressing your chest and abdomen using movement and simultaneously expanding them using breathing. This conflict between movement and breathing can adversely affect your health.

3. Do not move when holding the breath after inhalation. When the breath is held after inhalation, the chest and abdomen are fully expanded. The body offers maximum resistance to movement during this phase of the breathing cycle. Therefore, the breath should be held after inhalation only when you stay in a position, not during movement.

4. You can move when the breath is suspended after exhalation. When breathing is suspended after extended exhalation, the chest is completely relaxed and the abdomen is drawn inward. The body offers less resistance to movement in this position, and so forward-bending movements can be done during this phase of the breathing cycle.

These four rules for combining movement and breathing are summarized in figure 2.10.

Keep Your Breathing Deep and Effortless

One commentary on the *Yoga-Sutras* defines the most important quality of an asana in one word: natural. To derive maximum benefit from doing an asana, it must be natural, effortless; we must be completely comfortable, at ease, in it. Only when we are truly comfortable in an asana can we breathe naturally—smoothly, deeply, and freely. Only when we breathe like this in the asana will we derive the benefit envisioned in the ancient

texts: the maintenance or restoration of optimal flow of *prana*, or, in simpler terms, the optimal functioning of our body and mind.

If we force ourselves into an asana, stress and discomfort will disturb our breathing. As a consequence, we will certainly develop imbalances in our body and mind. This is totally contrary to the spirit behind the practice of yoga as a whole. A body position that disturbs your breathing is not an asana. Never sacrifice the quality of your breathing to attain the form of an asana. This will defeat the purpose of asana practice.

Keep Your Spine Strong and Flexible

In order for you to inhale deeply, the chest must expand fully. In order for you to exhale deeply, the abdominal muscles must contract. Therefore, for you to do full and deep breathing with ease, complete movement of the chest and abdomen are necessary. Strength, flexibility, and proper alignment of the trunk are essential for deep and free breathing. The spine forms the central axis of the trunk. Therefore, to do proper breathing, it is vital that we keep our spine in good shape.

DEVELOPING STRENGTH, FLEXIBILITY, AND STRUCTURAL ALIGNMENT

Asanas can provide structural, functional, and psychological benefits. The principal structural benefits are strength, flexibility, and proper body alignment or symmetry. How do

1 **Do these movements on inhalation:**

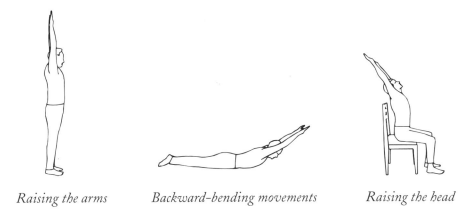

Raising the arms   *Backward-bending movements*   *Raising the head*

2 **Do these movements on exhalation:**

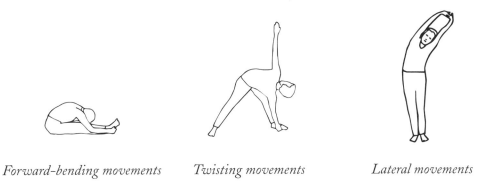

Forward-bending movements   *Twisting movements*   *Lateral movements*

3 **Do not move when holding the breath after inhalation.**

4 **You can move when the breath is suspended after exhalation.**

Fig. 2.10. The four rules for combining movement and breathing.

we determine the structural benefit of an asana? Will an asana increase strength or flexibility? Can one asana do both? What types of asanas can help in maintaining or correcting alignment?

To answer these questions, we need to understand how the components of an asana are related to the three goals of strength, flexibility, and structural alignment. That is, we need to know what types of movements or body positions, done with appropriate breathing, can give us each of these benefits.

Strength

When our muscles repeatedly contract with more force than they are normally used to exerting, their strength increases over time. Therefore, to increase the strength of our muscles using asanas, we have to do movements or stay in positions in which our muscles contract strongly or at least with more force than in our daily activities. Usually, in asana practice, we lift some part of the body against the force of gravity to increase strength. We can, of course, use external weights if greater strengthening is required (figs. 2.11, 2.12, 2.13).

Flexibility

To increase flexibility, we need to stretch our muscles and other connective tissues. In asanas, movements that go with gravity and those that go against gravity can stretch the body and thus increase flexibility. However, it is often convenient to use the force of gravity to assist in stretching the body (figs. 2.14, 2.15).

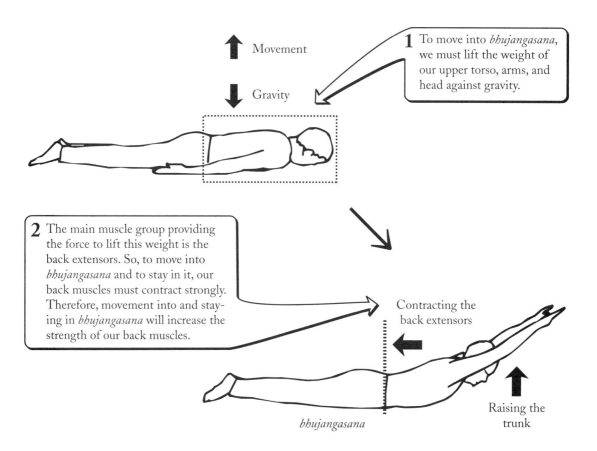

Movement

Gravity

1 To move into *bhujangasana*, we must lift the weight of our upper torso, arms, and head against gravity.

2 The main muscle group providing the force to lift this weight is the back extensors. So, to move into *bhujangasana* and to stay in it, our back muscles must contract strongly. Therefore, movement into and staying in *bhujangasana* will increase the strength of our back muscles.

Contracting the back extensors

bhujangasana

Raising the trunk

Fig. 2.11. Movement into and staying in *bhujangasana* strengthens the back muscles.

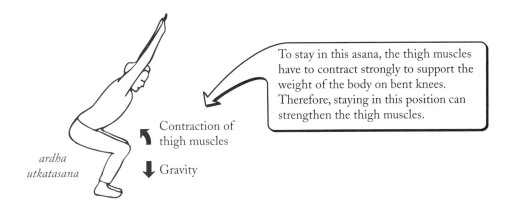

Fig. 2.12. Staying in *ardha utkatasana* strengthens the thigh muscles.

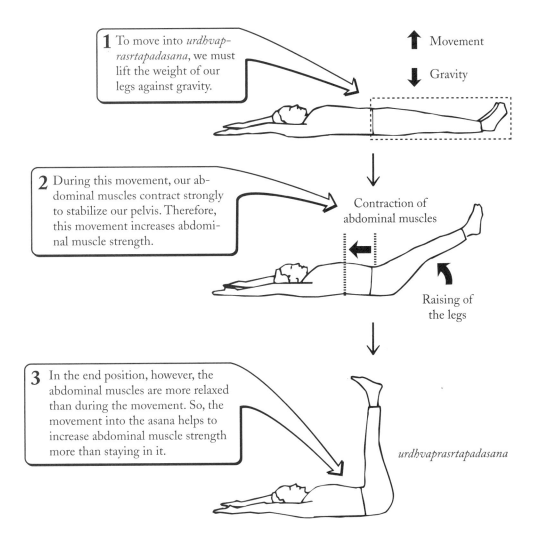

Fig. 2.13. Movement into *urdhvaprasrtapadasana* strengthens the abdominal muscles.

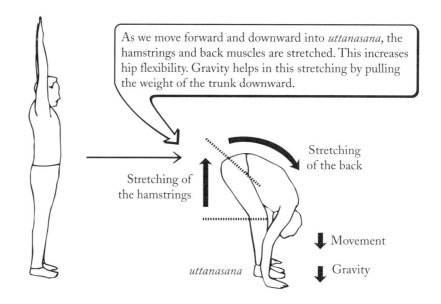

As we move forward and downward into *uttanasana*, the hamstrings and back muscles are stretched. This increases hip flexibility. Gravity helps in this stretching by pulling the weight of the trunk downward.

Stretching of the back

Stretching of the hamstrings

↓ Movement

↓ Gravity

uttanasana

Fig. 2.14. Movement into and staying in *uttanasana* increases hip flexibility.

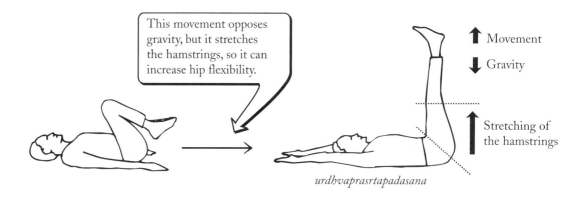

This movement opposes gravity, but it stretches the hamstrings, so it can increase hip flexibility.

↑ Movement

↓ Gravity

↑ Stretching of the hamstrings

urdhvaprasrtapadasana

Fig. 2.15. Movement into and staying in *urdhvaprasrtapadasana* also increases hip flexibility.

Alignment

Asanas can make a valuable contribution to our health by helping to maintain or restore our body's proper structural alignment. In today's world, both the workplace and many sporting activities promote structural mis-alignment in our body. Tennis, for example, requires continuous, strenuous use of one side of the body, while the other side remains rela-tively unused. Other sports like football or soccer also use one side of the body more than the other. Even symmetrical exercises like jogging and swimming can aggravate latent structural imbalances in our body because we usually unconsciously emphasize one side more than the other. Consequently, few forms of exercise are useful in correcting existing structural misalignments.

Asanas, however, are very useful in pre-venting and correcting structural imbalances in the body (fig. 2.16).

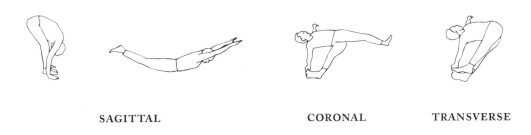

SAGITTAL　　　　**CORONAL**　　　**TRANSVERSE**

using the full range of movement in all three axes.

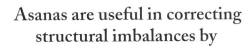

**Asanas are useful in correcting
structural imbalances by**

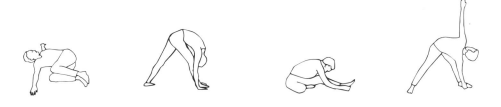

using movements to work on each side of the body separately.

Fig. 2.16. Asanas offer useful tools for correcting structural misalignments.

Misalignment is the abnormal positioning of some body part. It may occur in one or more of the three axes. In asanas we have movements in all three planes available to us. This allows us to work effectively with misalignments of body parts along any axis (see chapter 3).

More important, many movements in asanas are asymmetrical—they work separately with the two sides of the body. We repeat the movement a number of times, first on one side and then the other. All twisting and lateral movements and some forward- and backward-bending movements are asymmetrical. Further, many symmetrical forward- and backward-bending movements can be made asymmetrical by altering the position of the arms and legs before or during the movement. Using variations on this theme, we can design specific, effective exercises for correcting all types of body misalignment (for examples, see the case studies on scoliosis in chapter 8).

THE IMPORTANCE OF THE SPINE

The Structural Axis

The spine forms the central axis in the human body. To describe the structure of the human body in the simplest terms, we can say that we have a central trunk to which are attached two lower limbs (legs), two upper limbs (arms), and the head. The important skeletal elements of the trunk are the pelvis at the lower end and the shoulder girdle at the upper end. The two are connected by the central vertebral column, on top of which rests the head.

Our spine can move in all three planes: It is capable of flexion and extension, lateral movement, and rotation. In fact, such movements of the spine are inherent in all our normal activities because movements of all body parts—the arms, legs, head, and trunk—have an effect on the shape of the spine. For example, to walk, we need to raise our legs off the floor alternately. The simple movement of raising one leg off the floor causes the pelvis to tilt. This exerts a pull on the spine, causing it to bend to one side. Such movement of the spine is necessary to allow free and complete movement of other parts of the body. Therefore, strength, flexibility, and especially proper alignment of the spine are vital in maintaining sound body structure.

The spine is also linked with the physiology of body systems and the functioning of the mind. The spine forms the central support for the trunk, and the trunk contains most of the body's important organs. Also, spinal nerves supplying most of the body emerge from between the spinal vertebrae. Therefore, structural misalignment of the vertebral column can disturb the functioning of various body systems.

The shape of our spine is also related to our mental state. Our spine straightens when our mind is attentive and slumps when our mind is dull. Breathing is also linked with the shape of our spine. For example, when we inhale deeply in the chest, the curvature of our upper back is flattened.

Ancient yoga texts emphasize the importance of maintaining the structure of the spine. They express the distance between the important centers of the spine in terms of *angula*s (an individualized measure of distance based on the width of a person's finger) and stress the need to maintain these distances.

Movements of the body and breathing patterns affect the spine. In asana practice, we use the appropriate movements with breathing to maintain the spine's strength and flexibility. We will discuss how to do this in greater detail later. First let us look into the structure of the spine.

The Curvatures of the Spine

The spine has four curvatures, three of which change with body movement and breathing. The spine is straight when viewed from the front or the back. Viewed from the side, it has four curvatures. From the top down, they are as follows:

1. The cervical curvature, concave posteriorly
2. The thoracic curvature, convex posteriorly
3. The lumbar curvature, concave posteriorly
4. The sacral curvature, convex posteriorly

Of these four curvatures, the sacral curvature is fixed because the sacral vertebrae are fused. The other three curvatures (cervical, thoracic, and lumbar) are flexible: They can increase or decrease with movements of the body and with breathing. The lumbar and cervical curvatures are similar in shape (concave posteriorly), while the thoracic curvature has the opposite shape (convex posteriorly) (fig. 2.17). You can easily feel these curvatures in your back; they are similar to those of your spine. This is why, when we look at someone's back, the upper back is convex toward us, while the lower back and the neck are concave or hollow.

The curvatures of the spine should be maintained without increase or decrease. You might have noticed that the adjacent curvatures of the spine are opposite in shape. This characteristic allows them to support each other. Like inhalation and exhalation, they do not oppose but complement each other. The

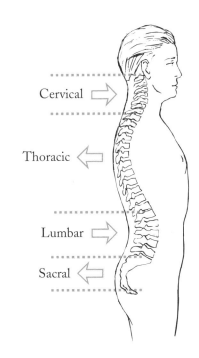

Fig. 2.17. The curvatures of the spine. The adjacent curvatures of the spine are opposite, yet they do not oppose but support each other.

curvatures of the spine are integral to its strength. So, to maintain the strength and flexibility of your spine, you must maintain its curvatures. That is why we attach such importance to the curvatures of the spine and the relationship between them when designing an asana program.

Unfortunately, the curvatures of our spine do not remain intact as we age. As we grow older, all the curvatures of the spine tend to increase: The shoulders become rounded and stooped (increase in thoracic curvature); the head is lifted to look forward (increase in cervical curvature); and the abdomen bulges out (increase in lumbar curvature). This change in the shape of the spine is due to the continued influence of gravity and a progressive decline in muscle strength and tone, accelerated by decreased use of some muscle groups.

Asana practice, using appropriate movements and breathing, can prevent or offset this tendency of the spine to slump with aging. Therefore, in asanas, we try to straighten both the lower and upper back, decreasing both their curvatures. The aim is not to decrease the curvatures of the spine to less than normal but to prevent them from increasing to more than the ideal (fig. 2.18).

When evaluating or designing any asana practice, we must consider the effect it has on the spine. If we disregard this important consideration, it is easy to arrive at a practice that may increase both structural and functional imbalance.

MAXIMIZING THE BENEFITS OF MOVEMENT AND BREATHING

Since adjacent segments of the spine have opposite curvatures, particular movements and breathing have a similar effect on the curvatures of the neck and lower back but an opposite effect on the curvature of the upper back. That is, movements and breathing that reduce the curvature (flatten the convexity) of the upper back usually increase the curvature (deepen the concavity) of the lower back and neck, and vice versa.

We may want only one of these effects and not the other. Therefore, we must use techniques that will maximize the beneficial effect of the movement or component of the breathing cycle on the spine while keeping the unwanted effect to a minimum.

Breathing

Correct breathing is of critical importance in working effectively with the spine. It is one of the important reasons for the success of asanas in correcting spinal problems. The techniques of breathing explained below are the key to using breathing to benefit the spine and to support movement in asanas.

1. Make the exhalation long, with an emphasis on abdominal muscle contraction. Start the exhalation in the lower abdomen and move upward to the chest. As we have already seen, conscious extended exhalation with abdominal muscle contraction helps to

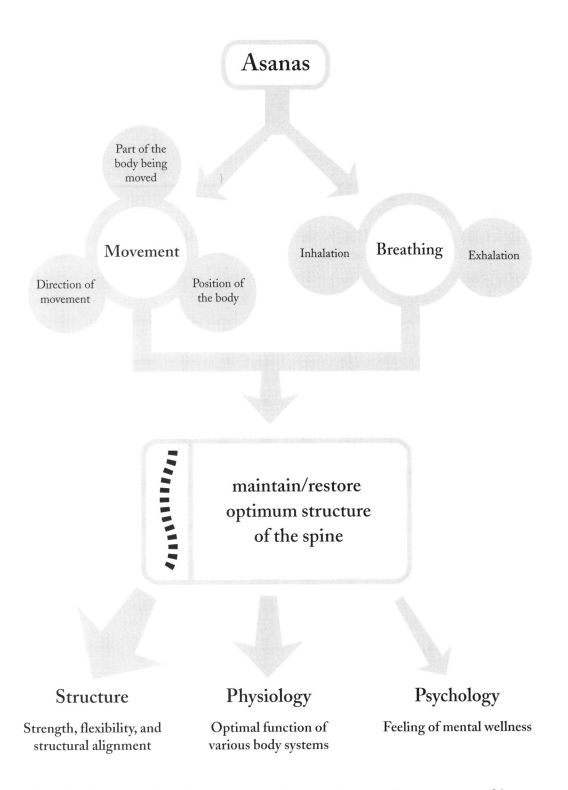

Fig. 2.18. Movement and breathing in asanas should restore and maintain the proper structure of the spine. This will positively affect our structure, function, and psychology.

prevent an increase in the curvature of the lower back. But it also collapses the chest and rounds the upper back. To keep the spine in good shape, we should emphasize the first effect and minimize the second.

To do this, you should exhale as follows: Begin exhalation with a contraction of the lower part of your abdomen. As you exhale further, allow the upper part of your abdomen to move in as well. Allow your chest to relax and collapse completely only as you reach the end of exhalation.

2. Make the inhalation deep, with an emphasis on expanding the chest. Start the inhalation in the chest and move downward to the abdomen. As we have seen, deep inhalation, with an emphasis on expanding the chest, straightens the curvature of the upper back. But it also deepens the curvature of the lower back and pushes the abdomen outward. We want to maximize the first effect and minimize the second.

To do this, you should inhale as follows: Start by allowing your chest to expand, straightening your upper back as much possible. As this happens, gradually relax your abdominal muscles that were contracted during exhalation, allowing your abdomen to move outward from the top downward. Your lower abdomen should move outward only as you near the end of inhalation.

Movement

Below we discuss the effect of the common types of movements seen in asanas on the back and the curvatures of the spine, followed by techniques for maximizing the benefit of these movements. You can observe these changes in the shape of the spine when another person does these movements. However, it is important to feel these changes in the shape of your own spine by doing these simple movements, because being aware of the effect of asanas on the spine as you do them can significantly enhance the quality of your practice.

Use forward-bending movements to stretch your back and flatten the curvature of your lower back. Forward-bending movements are similar to exhalation in their effect on the spine. When we bend forward, our upper back is rounded and our shoulders tend to slump. But the curvature of our lower back is flattened, and the back is stretched (fig. 2.19). Forward-bending movements done from the standing, seated, and lying body positions all have this effect (fig. 2.20). In the lying position, instead of bending our trunk forward, over our legs, we move our legs toward the trunk. The effect, however, is similar.

Forward-bending movements help to stretch our back and prevent our lower back curvature from increasing. This is the positive effect that forward-bending movements can have on our spine.

We do not want our upper back to be rounded or our shoulders and upper spine to slump. But these are the two unwanted effects of forward-bending movements on our back and spine.

The following techniques will help you maximize stretching your spine in forward-

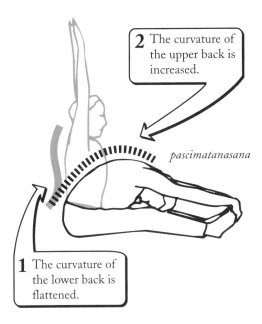

2 The curvature of the upper back is increased.

pascimatanasana

1 The curvature of the lower back is flattened.

Fig. 2.19. Changes in the shape of the spine in *pascimatanasana*, a seated forward-bending asana.

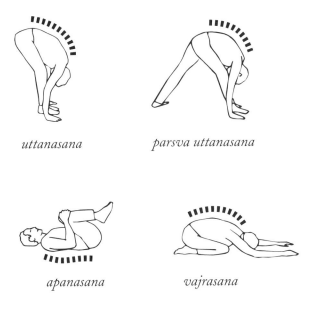

uttanasana

parsva uttanasana

apanasana

vajrasana

Fig. 2.20. Changes in the shape of the spine in other forward-bending asanas. The change is similar to what occurs in *pascimatanasana*, as shown in figure 2.19. Note that in *apanasana*, the legs are brought toward the trunk, while in the others, the trunk is folded over the legs.

bending movements, without rounding your upper back and shoulders more than necessary.

To maximize the benefit of forward-bending movements, do the following:

- Reach out as you do the forward-bending movements. Consciously try to stretch your back. For example, when you bend downward and forward into *uttanasana*, try to stretch and reach forward, as if you are trying to touch an object just beyond your fingers (fig. 2.21).
- Actively extend your spine (arch your back) when you make the movement out of the asana. Done in this manner, the return movement can be an effective backward-bending movement in some asanas like *uttanasana*. By doing this, you will be doing a forward-bending as well as a backward-bending movement in the same asana, though the forward-bending movement will be the more intense of the two (fig. 2.22).
- Keep your head down. Forward-bending movements are useful for stretching not only the back but also the neck. In forward-bending movements, the back is rounded and the spine is curved forward. The curvature of the neck should be in line with the rest of the spine. If you do not lower your head, you will create stress in your neck, shoulders, and upper back.

Use backward-bending movements to strengthen your back and decrease the curvature of your upper back. The effect of

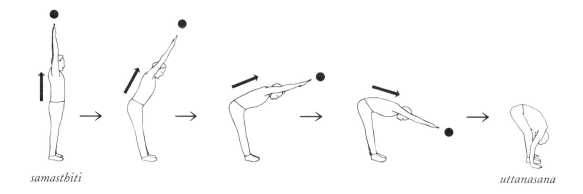

samasthiti   *uttanasana*

Fig. 2.21. As you move into *uttanasana*, stretch forward, as if you are trying to touch the black spot.

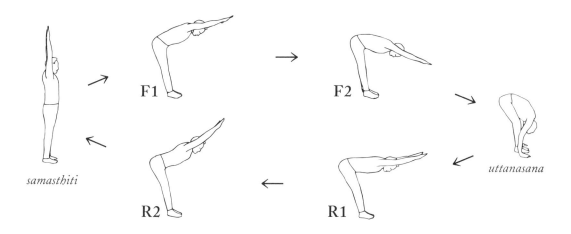

samasthiti   *uttanasana*

Fig. 2.22. Compare the shape of the back in the corresponding positions (F1 and R2, F2 and R1) during the movement into and out of *uttanasana*. Note how arching or extending the back during the return movement makes it similar to a mild backward-bending movement.

backward-bending movements on the spine is similar to that of inhalation. When we bend our trunk backward, the curvature of our lower back increases. Our upper back is straightened, and its curvature is flattened (figs. 2.23, 2.24).

To do backward-bending movements, our back muscles have to contract. Also, in many backward-bending asanas, the movement is done against gravity, which adds to the effort required from our back muscles. Therefore, backward-bending movements can strengthen our back.

Backward-bending movements strengthen our back muscles and straighten our upper back. These are two important positive effects of backward-bending movements on our back and spine.

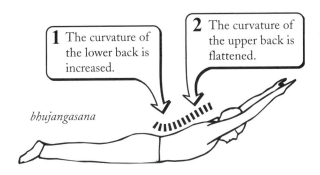

Fig. 2.23. Change in the shape of the spine in *bhujangasana*: a lying backward-bending asana.

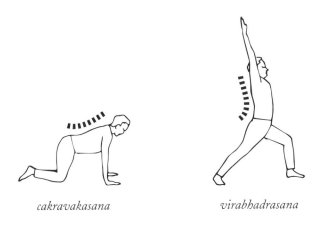

Fig. 2.24. Change in the shape of the spine in two other common backward-bending asanas, one from the kneeling position and the other from the standing position. The change is similar to that in *bhujangasana*.

We do not want our lower back curvature to increase, but we cannot avoid this happening in backward-bending movements. This is the unwanted effect of backward-bending movements on the spine.

The following techniques help to maximize the straightening of the upper back and the strengthening of the back without hollowing the lower back too much.

To maximize the benefit of backward-bending movements, do the following:

- Consciously emphasize the extension of your upper back and avoid compressing your lower back. Try not to compress your lower back when you arch into the backward bend. Instead, as with forward-bending movements, try to reach out and stretch as you arch your back (fig. 2.25). Use the inhalation to expand your chest and support the extension of your upper back.
- Keep your neck in line with your spine. Raising your head will accentuate the hollowing of your lower back, which you do not want; it may even lead to a headache because of the stress it creates in the region of the neck (fig. 2.26).

Use twisting movements to rotate the spine. Twisting movements, apart from their use in correcting structural misalignments, are useful in rotating the spine. To twist or rotate the spine, try to keep one end of the trunk fixed and rotate the other end. The rotation of the spine takes place around an axis extending vertically through it. In standing and seated twists, we keep our hips and the lower part of our trunk fixed and rotate the upper end of our trunk and our head. In lying twists, we keep the upper end of our trunk relatively immobile and rotate the lower part of the trunk and our legs. In the spine itself, most rotation takes place in the thoracic and cervical regions. The lumbar spine cannot rotate much.

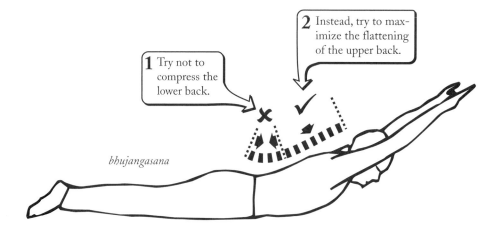

Fig. 2.25. Technique to maximize the positive effect of backward-bending asanas on the spine.

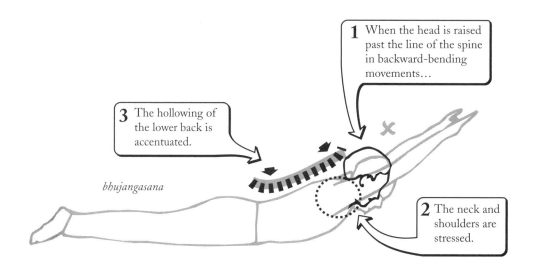

Fig. 2.26. Do not raise your head past the line of your spine in backward-bending asanas.

To maximize the benefit of twisting movements, assess how much the moving end of the trunk is rotated relative to the fixed end. The appearance of the asana may not be an accurate guide to the intensity of the twisting movement. When gauging the intensity of twisting in an asana, do not judge by how much the entire trunk is rotated.

In seated twisting movements, the hips are almost completely immobile, and the lower trunk is relatively fixed. Only the upper part of trunk—the shoulders, arms, and head—

can rotate (fig. 2.27). In comparison, in a standing twisting movement, the entire trunk, including the hips, can rotate to some extent (fig. 2.28).

You can turn the trunk more in a standing position than in a seated position, especially when the feet are together. But the effect of the twisting movement on the spine is more intense in the seated position. The true marker of the intensity of the twisting movement is the degree to which one end of the trunk turns with reference to the other end. Therefore, turning the entire trunk is like rolling to one side, not twisting.

Do not lean to the side of the twist. This can make the twisting movement appear more intense while compromising its effectiveness. Try to keep the other side of your body pressed down firmly, distributing your weight as evenly as possible (fig. 2.29).

Use arm movements to work on your upper back. When we raise our arms, our upper back is straightened to some extent, and our chest opens out. Simultaneously, the curvature of our lower back increases slightly. That is, raising our arms affects our spine like a mild backward-bending movement (fig. 2.30).

You can clearly feel the hollowing of your lower back as you raise your arms, if you do it when lying on your back with your legs stretched out. This is because this body position—supine with the legs stretched out—itself increases the curvature of the lower back to some extent. In fact, in some therapeutic situations, such as low back pain, simple arm

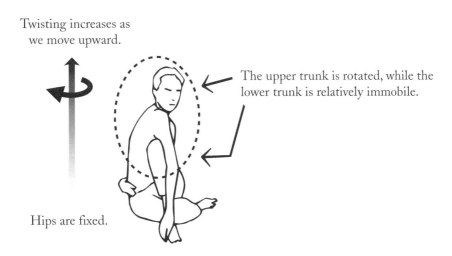

Twisting increases as we move upward.

The upper trunk is rotated, while the lower trunk is relatively immobile.

Hips are fixed.

Fig. 2.27. An example of a twisting movement from the seated position (*ardha matsyendrasana*). The hips are relatively straight, with the most twisting taking place in the upper part of the body.

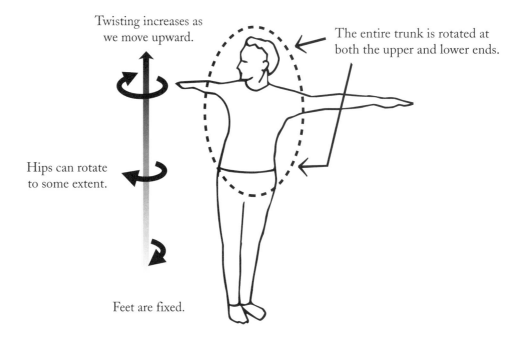

Twisting increases as
we move upward.

The entire trunk is rotated at
both the upper and lower ends.

Hips can rotate
to some extent.

Feet are fixed.

Fig. 2.28. Twisting from the standing position in *samasthiti*.

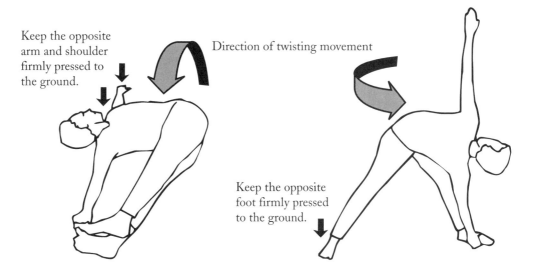

Keep the opposite
arm and shoulder
firmly pressed to
the ground.

Direction of twisting movement

Keep the opposite
foot firmly pressed
to the ground.

Fig. 2.29. To maximize the effect of a twisting movement, do not lean to the side of the twist.

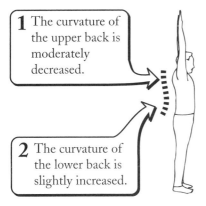

1 The curvature of the upper back is moderately decreased.

2 The curvature of the lower back is slightly increased.

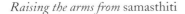

Raising the arms from samasthiti

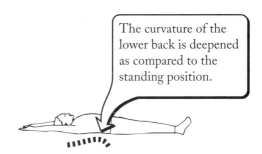

The curvature of the lower back is deepened as compared to the standing position.

Raising the arms from savasana

Fig. 2.30. The effect of raising the arms on the curvatures of the spine, when done from standing and lying positions.

raising from the lying position can serve as a backward-bending movement.

Raising the arms is very important to effectively straighten the upper back, expand the chest, and support full inhalation. That is why most trunk movements in asanas are done with raised arms, whatever the direction of the movement—forward, backward, twisting, or lateral. Arm movements can be used to get the best from both forward- and backward-bending movements.

To maximize the benefit of arm movements, do the following:

- Do not keep your arms stiff and rigid. Relax your elbows and wrists slightly and stretch from your trunk and shoulders.
- When you move into a forward bend, use your arms to help stretch your back. Keeping your arms raised will also help to limit the rounding of the upper back that occurs with this movement.

- Keep your arms in line with your spine, in both forward- and backward-bending movements (fig. 2.31). Raising your arms as you do backward-bending movements is useful in supporting the work on the upper back and shoulders and in increasing the extension of the spine. But if you raise your arms before your trunk, it will stress your shoulders, upper back, and neck.
- When you move out of a forward bend, use your arms to help extend your spine.

Use leg movements to work on your lower back. As we have seen, lying on the back with the legs stretched out deepens the curvature of the lower back. If the legs are bent at the knees, the curvature of the lower back is flattened, and the abdominal muscles are relaxed. Because of this, many people find this position more comfortable than lying down with the legs straight. Therefore, this is a good position in which to do relaxation breathing.

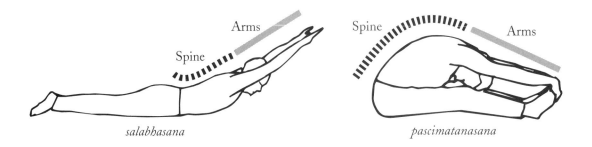

salabhasana   *pascimatanasana*

Fig. 2.31. The arms should be in line with the spine in both forward- and backward-bending movements.

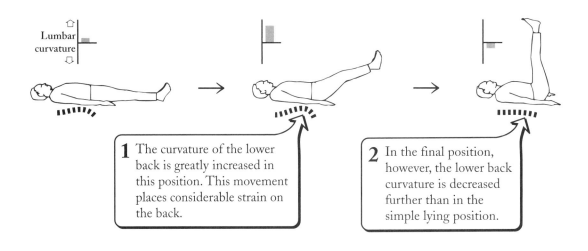

Lumbar curvature

1 The curvature of the lower back is greatly increased in this position. This movement places considerable strain on the back.

2 In the final position, however, the lower back curvature is decreased further than in the simple lying position.

Fig. 2.32. The effect on the spine of raising the legs from the supine position, while keeping them straight.

Spreading the legs tends to increase the curvature of the lower back in all body positions: standing, seated, lying, and inverted.

Raising the legs in the lying position, while keeping them straight, has a strong effect on the lower back. The lower back is placed under considerable stress and the curvature may increase, especially at the start of the movement. As the legs are raised further, the stress on the lower back gradually decreases, and in the final position, the curvature of the lower back is flattened (fig. 2.32).

USING BREATHING TO MAXIMIZE THE BENEFIT OF MOVEMENT

Breathing is the key to intensifying the effect of movement into or staying in asanas. When you stay in asanas, gradually try to move deeper into the asana during the supporting component of the breathing cycle. During the other component of the breathing cycle, relax a little. If you do this, you can set up a cycle of alternate effort and relaxation, of work and rest. This is an intelligent method of moving deeper into the asana, without stressing your body (fig. 2.33).

For example, in an asana like *uttanasana*, stretch and move deeper into the forward bend on exhalation. On inhalation, allow yourself to relax a little. Stretch again, a little more if possible, on the next exhalation, and so on. In backward bends like *salabhasana*, increase your effort—raise your trunk and legs a little more—with each inhalation. On each exhalation, relax and allow your trunk and legs to move down a little.

Even when you have enough strength or flexibility to move into the asana completely, this slight movement with breathing is very important. To avoid stressing your body, you should not make staying in asanas a static, rigid exercise. If you use breathing in this way, there will be subtle, deep movement even when you stay in asanas.

Another reason you should use this technique is to maximize the flow of breathing and minimize the conflict between the body position and your breathing. If your trunk is fully bent forward, as in *uttanasana*, you naturally cannot inhale as easily as you can exhale. If you allow your trunk to lift a little with each inhalation, you can breathe in a little more deeply and with less difficulty. As a natural consequence, your next exhalation will be longer and deeper, for you cannot breathe out unless you breathe in (and vice versa).

In a backward-bending asana like *salabhasana*, the body will naturally move down a little on exhalation, because inhalation and the expansion of the chest are supporting the body

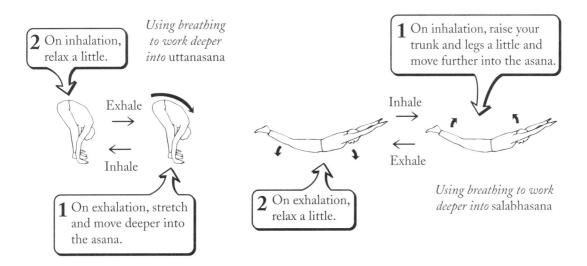

Fig. 2.33. Using breathing to work deeper into an asana.

to some extent. If you try to maintain the body position rigidly during exhalation, you will be straining yourself unnecessarily. If you wish to make your practice more demanding, it is better to relax and allow yourself to move down a little during exhalation, and put your effort into raising your chest and legs more on the next inhalation. That way, breathing and movement will go together, as they naturally should. Keep in mind that your breathing should always be smooth and controlled. Your effort should be as well. If your movement is jerky or your breathing short, shallow, or disturbed, you are forcing yourself into the asana, not intelligently working into it. You may need to rest or simply give yourself more time for preparation.

Further details on using breathing effectively in asana practice are given in my book *Yoga for Body, Breath, and Mind* (Shambhala Publications, 2002).

IMPROVING THE FUNCTION OF BODY SYSTEMS

Ancient yoga texts view disease as an imbalance in the flow of prana, or life force, in the body. The breath is considered to be linked to the flow of prana and is therefore very important in restoring the flow of prana, or proper functioning, to affected body systems. Therefore, the approach of yoga to the therapy of disorders of body function is critically dependent on the proper use of breathing. The role of movement alone in

correcting functional disorders is relatively limited; breathing plays the key role. We will discuss the concept of prana and the role of breathing in greater detail in chapters 5, 6, and 7.

ACHIEVING MENTAL STEADINESS

Classical texts on yoga, such as the *Hatha-Yoga-Pradipika*, state that the most important aim of the practice of asanas is to reduce rajas and tamas in the mind and to reinforce sattva. In other words, asanas should increase our mental calm and clarity. This is the key feature of asanas that sets them apart from all other forms of exercise.

Mental Focus

To increase our mental steadiness, we need to focus our mind. In time, this will reduce our mind's tendency toward distraction and bring about awareness and quietness. This is the basis of the practice of meditation. Asana can itself be a form of meditation.

An approach with universal applicability that also exploits the natural connection between our body, breath, and mind is to focus our mind on the movement of our body or on the flow of our breath during the practice of asanas. Other forms of mental focus can also be incorporated in asanas, but here we primarily discuss this very effective technique that everyone can use.

Focusing on the Breath

It is better to focus your mind on your breathing than on your movement. The reason is this: Breathing has a natural involuntary pattern. To make your breathing longer and smoother or of a specific duration, it is essential that your mind be constantly aware of the flow of your breath. If your mind wanders and your awareness fades, your breathing will slip back to its usual involuntary pattern. This will alert you to the lack of focus in your mind and allow you to regain it.

Movement, on the other hand, has no natural involuntary pattern. Patterns of movement that we do consciously can be learned over time. The patterns of movement that we do in asanas can also be learned, just as we learn to swim or ride a bicycle. Therefore, any asana program, no matter how varied the movements are, can become a mechanical exercise that can be done very well with minimal attention. In other words, most patterns or sequences of movement can be "programmed" so that they can be done with little conscious attention or with only intermittent attention. Breathing cannot be programmed in this way. Therefore, if you wish to see when your mind is wandering, observing movement is not as useful as observing breathing.

Containing Movement within Breathing

When you move into or out of any asana, begin the breathing first and then begin to move. When the movement ends, your breath should continue for a short while, perhaps two to three seconds (fig. 2.34).

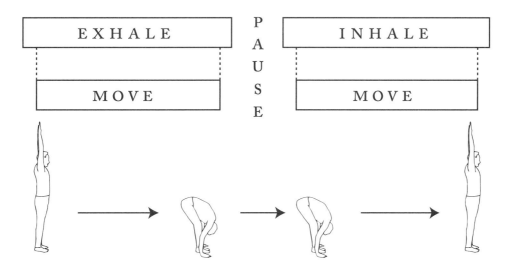

Fig. 2.34. Movement must always be contained within breathing when practicing asanas.

Physically, this technique serves two important purposes: One, it minimizes the possibility of an inadvertent conflict between movement and breathing. Because we begin to breathe before we move, we do not move when the breath is held—which would create conflict between breathing and movement. For example, when we do *uttanasana*, we first raise our arms and inhale fully. Then we begin to bend down. If we exhale a little and then begin bending forward, it will minimize the resistance that a fully expanded chest and abdomen might offer to movement.

Two, breathing before movement maximizes the support that breathing extends to movement. For example, in *bhujangasana*, if we begin inhaling first, it will expand our chest and make the movement of raising our trunk and arms easier.

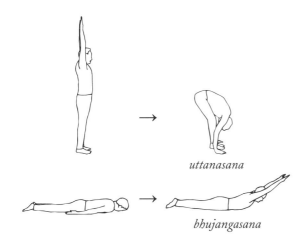

uttanasana

bhujangasana

The most important benefit of this technique, however, is the effect it can have on our mind. Doing breathing and movement together may seem ideal, but it is not, especially because of its effect on our mental focus. As we have seen, it is better to focus our mind on observing and directing the flow of our breathing because of its variable and inherently unprogrammable rhythm.

Initiating and terminating each cycle of breathing in sync with movement makes adhering to a particular breathing rhythm a semiautomatic act because of the partly subconscious nature of the movement. That is, if you begin and end movement and breathing simultaneously, you will end up allowing the movements to direct the rhythm of your breathing cycle instead of using mental focus to do this.

This technique sounds rather simple, but its effect is profound. You must practice it to understand how important it is. Try following it carefully in an asana practice of just half an hour. You will see that it is almost impossible to maintain the continuous mental focus required to ensure that the movement is always contained within breathing.

The nature of this technique ensures that it will not become mechanical. It is also useful in helping us to assess our mental focus when we practice asanas. On the days when you are able to focus your mind well, you will see that there is considerably greater quietness and calm in your mind following your asana practice.

THE BIOMECHANICS OF ASANAS

One strength of the approach of asanas is its simplicity. Classical texts on yoga follow a practical and experiential approach, not a biomechanical one. The same is largely true of this book as well. You can observe all the principles we outline in your own body, breath, and mind during your practice or by trying the movements and breathing techniques we have suggested as examples. However, a high level of awareness is required.

Understanding a few simple biomechanical concepts and how they apply to the practice of asanas can help you design more effective asana programs. To use these ideas effectively, however, it is important that you do the movements and feel how these principles translate into practice, because these instructions consist largely of experiential knowledge explained in technical language. As you become more familiar with the movements in asanas and their effects, these principles will recede to the back of your mind and you will develop the ability to naturally and instinctively judge the effects of combinations of movements and their applications to particular individuals and conditions.

Gravity and Muscle Contraction

Asanas combine movement and breathing. Our body moves when a force is applied to it. In asanas, we need to consider two forces: first, gravity, and second, the force generated by the contraction of our own muscles. The interplay of these two forces determines the body's movements.

Gravity is a constant external force pulling us downward. Muscles generate forces in our body. Muscles are responsible for most movements that occur in our various body systems.

Our heart pumping blood, food moving through our intestines, and the maintenance of blood pressure by our blood vessels all happen because of muscular contraction, but the contraction of these muscles is not under our conscious control. We cannot, for instance, decide to propel the food in our intestines faster or keep it waiting for an hour or two! Once we have swallowed our food, the subsequent processes are largely involuntary.

In contrast, the movements of our head, trunk, and limbs are under our control. This is because the contraction of the muscles responsible for their movement can be initiated by us at will. The movements we do in asanas, and in fact all movements we make in our daily life, are a consequence of the contraction of these voluntary muscles. When we perform a movement, we are ordering the muscles responsible for that movement to contract, even though this may not always be reflected in our conscious perception. Since the movements we make in asanas are voluntary, this discussion will be limited to voluntary muscles (skeletal muscles) and their relation to forces and movement.

Muscles generate force only by contraction. Muscles can only pull, not push. That is, they can generate force only by shortening, not by expanding or lengthening. An increase in the length of a muscle is not due to the force generated within it. A force external to the muscle, pulling the muscle at one or both ends, is necessary to stretch the muscle. In our bodies, the force required to stretch a muscle is provided by gravity or by the contraction of other muscles.

Also, when a muscle contracts, it exerts force at both its ends, pulling them toward each other. Which end will move depends on their relative fixity.

Lever Systems

So far, we have seen that gravity and muscle contraction are the two forces responsible for movement of the body and that muscles generate force by shortening. The next question is, how is force translated into movement in the body?

Most movements of the body skeleton are accomplished through a system of levers. A lever basically consists of a bar or rod, or any rigid object, which is fixed at one point. When a force is applied at any other point along its length, the object rotates around the fixed point. This point around which the rotation takes place is the fulcrum. The force is usually termed the effort, and the weight to be moved or lifted is called the load. The load may be just the weight of the object itself, or there may be some other added weight as well. There are innumerable examples of the application of levers in our daily life—doors, crowbars, and forceps, to name a few.

There are three orders of levers, depending on the position of the effort and load in relation to the fulcrum. In levers of the first order, the fulcrum is between the effort and load (E-F-L). In levers of the second order, the load is between the effort and fulcrum (E-L-F). In levers of the third order, the effort is between the fulcrum and the load (F-E-L).

In our body, bones form the bars—the rigid components of the lever system. Muscles are attached to bones, and they exert a pulling force on the bone at the point of their attachment. This is the effort. The load is the weight of the body part, along with any external weights attached to it and any resistance to the movement. The fulcrum is the joint around which the rotary movement of the bone takes place.

In the body, most lever systems are of the third order. The point of attachment of the muscle on the bone (the point of application of effort) is relatively close to the joint (fulcrum). A larger portion of the limb or body part, and consequently the center of gravity that determines the position of the load, is distal to the point of attachment of the muscle. In other words, the effort (the force generated by muscle contraction) is applied between the fulcrum (the joint) and the load (the weight of the body part).

For example, consider the elbow joint (fig. 2.35). The joint is the fulcrum. The bones of the forearm form the lever. The brachialis muscle provides the force to bend the elbow. This muscle extends from the bone of the upper arm to the bones of the forearm, close to the elbow joint. To raise the forearm, the weight of the forearm and hand have to be lifted. This constitutes the load. The load can be considered to lie at the center of gravity of the forearm, which is roughly in its middle. Now, you can see that the load is at the middle of the forearm, while the effort is applied closer to the elbow. That is, the load is farther away from the fulcrum than the effort; in

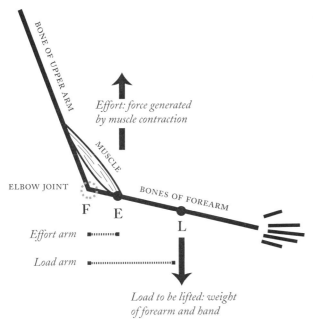

*Effort: force generated
by muscle contraction*

*Load to be lifted: weight
of forearm and hand*

Fig. 2.35. The lever system at the elbow joint. The fulcrum (F) is the elbow joint. The force is supplied by the muscle (brachialis) attached to the forearm bones at the point of application of effort (E). The load (L) is the weight of the forearm acting through the center of gravity of the forearm, situated approximately at the middle of its length. This is a lever system of the third order. The load arm is greater than the effort arm, and therefore the force exerted by the muscle must exceed the weight of the load.

other words, the effort arm is less than the load arm. Therefore, this is a lever of the third order.

In levers of the third order, the mechanical advantage is unfavorable. That is, the force applied is greater than the weight of the load lifted. But the load moves through a correspondingly greater distance than the point of application of the force moves. This is a compromise between strength and range of movement. The work done by the muscle is a

product of the force exerted and the distance through which it moves. If the load is placed closer to the fulcrum, less force is required to lift it, but it will move through a smaller distance. We can lift a greater weight if it is tied to the middle of our forearm than if it is tied to our hand, but the weight will move through a smaller distance.

Doors are common examples of this. A door is fixed to the frame at one side by hinges. The other side is free to rotate about the hinges. In this lever system, the hinges are the fulcrum and part of the weight of the door is the load. We apply force when we push the door. This force causes the door to rotate. The point where we place our hand is the point where the force or effort acts.

If our hand is close to the hinges, most of the door's weight will lie distal to our hand. In this case, the effort (hand) lies between the fulcrum (hinges) and the load (the rest of the door), so this is a lever system of third order. The mechanical advantage is unfavorable, and therefore opening a door in this way requires a lot of force—we have to push hard.

Conversely, if we push the door with our hand placed as far away from the hinge as possible, the effort required is minimal, as most of the door (load) is now between our hand (effort) and the hinges (fulcrum). This is an example of a lever of the second order, in which the mechanical advantage is favorable. This is how we normally open doors, and it is also why the handle on a door is usually placed far away from the hinges, close to the free end of the door.

Torque

A more accurate approach is to view the movements of the body in terms of torque, also called the moment of force. Torque is a measure of how much a force acting on an object causes it to rotate. As we have seen, body movements are generally due to the rotary movement of bones at joints. For instance, when we lift our leg, it does not separate from our body and move as a whole, like a stick being lifted off the ground. Instead, it rotates about one fixed end—the hip joint. As we have seen, bones move because muscle contraction exerts a force on them. Muscles exert a linear force at the point of their attachment to the bone. The amount of movement that this force will produce depends on the torque it exerts at the joint, and not just the magnitude of the force. The torque determines how much rotation the force elicits at the joint. Note that both load and effort are forces, though opposite in direction. We usually consider the weight of the body part or object to be the load, and the force exerted by us, the effort. To result in movement (rotation of the joint) in the direction of the effort, the torque exerted by the effort must exceed that exerted by the load.

A calculation of torque is needed to judge the effect of a change in the angle of application of force. Let us return to our example of a door. If we push the door with our hand placed at an oblique or acute angle to its surface, part of the force we apply will be used to pull the door away from its hinges or push it into them. The door will not rotate much,

and so this is an ineffective way of opening the door. This happens because the torque or amount of rotation elicited by a force is maximum when it is applied perpendicular to the surface of the object and decreases when the angle is greater or less than ninety degrees. This is reflected in our experience that the door can be moved with minimal effort when we push it with our arm directed perpendicular to its surface (with our palm flat on the door). This is the most efficient way to open a door and the way we do it naturally.

In the practice of asanas, the angle of application of force is of little importance, for the simple reason that it is not under our control. It is automatically decided by the position of body parts and the angle of insertion of the muscles into the bones. However, we need to keep this one point in mind: When the angle is either very small or very large, the linear forces being applied by the muscles on the bones and other connective tissue structures may be very high, though the torque produced will be minimal. As a consequence, the range and force of the rotary movement may be limited, but the stress on body structures will be considerable. That is, the force applied by the muscles is often much greater than the weight of the body part being lifted. Therefore, it is possible to place body structures under excessive strain inadvertently, especially when external weights are used.

A well-known illustration of this principle is how bending over from the hips to lift a large weight with the hands can result in damage to the intervertebral disks in the lumbar spine. In that position, the back extensors act at a highly unfavorable angle. Therefore, most of the force exerted by them translates into a linear compressive force acting along the length of the vertebral column, rather than the rotary force or torque required to lift the weight. This puts the intervertebral disks under great stress and can lead to low back pain.

In summary, most body movements are lever-type movements, with the joint as the fulcrum and the bones in the part being moved as the lever. The point of application of the force is the place where the muscle is inserted into the bone. Most lever systems in the body are of the third order, with the point of application of effort (muscle insertion) placed between the fulcrum (joint) and the load (the weight of the body parts distal to the point of muscle insertion). Therefore, the muscle usually has to contract with greater force than the weight of the load, as the effort arm is less than the load arm. The advantage of such an arrangement is that the decrease in the length of the muscle, as it shortens, is small; but the distance through which the body part moves is much greater. That is, the design of the human body sacrifices strength for a greater range of movement.

Levers in Asanas

In the body, we cannot change the point of attachment of muscles to the bones. That is, we cannot alter the point of application of the effort. The magnitude of the effort we make is determined by the load to be lifted. Therefore, in asanas, we primarily alter the amount of the load and the distance of the load from the joint. Though this happens naturally due to changes in body position, we can consciously use this to bring about specific changes in the effects of asanas.

Since the point of insertion of the muscles does not vary, and we are not looking into the complexities of changes brought about by joint movement, we only have to consider how the effort varies with change in the load. It should now be clear that the force we have to exert is not determined simply by the magnitude of the load but also by the distance of the load from the joint. The farther the load is from the joint, the greater the force needed to lift it. As we usually do not use external weights in asanas, the load we have to lift is only the weight of the body parts themselves.

Example 1: Consider the return movement from uttanasana *to* samasthiti, *or standing position* (fig. 2.36). The fulcrum in this movement is the hip joint. The weight of the arms and trunk is the load. The back extensors are the important muscle group providing the force required (effort). We require little effort to stay in *uttanasana* because in this position our body is mostly supported passively (by ligaments, muscle tension, and so on). In *uttanasana*, our trunk is very close to our legs and hips. As we return to the standing position, we raise our trunk, gradually moving it away from our legs and hips. The distance of our trunk from the line of our hips increases until the midway position (*ardha uttanasana*) and then gradually decreases as we return to the upright position. In the fully erect position

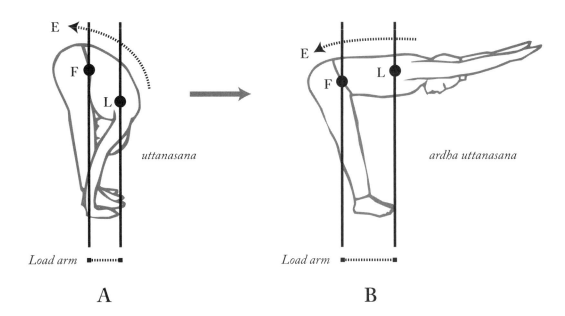

Fig. 2.36. In the return movement from *uttanasana* (A) to standing position, the halfway position is *ardha uttanasana* (B). The movement takes place about the fulcrum (F) lying approximately at the region of the hip joint. The load (L) is the weight of the trunk, head, and arms, acting through the common center of gravity (black circle). The force or effort (E) is provided mainly by the back and hip extensors. The perpendicular distance from the load to the fulcrum (load arm) is maximum in *ardha uttanasana*. Therefore, maximum effort is needed in this position.

(*samasthiti* with arms raised), our trunk is directly above our hips.

At all times, the force of muscle contraction has to exceed or at least match the load exerted by the weight of the trunk (the force exerted by the downward pull of gravity on the trunk). Only then will our trunk move upward, or at least remain where it is without descending. Also, as we have discussed, the effort required is greatest when the load is farthest away from the fulcrum. That is, the effort increases with increase in length of the load arm. In the movement from *uttanasana* to *samasthiti*, the load arm is longest when our trunk is farthest from our hips. This happens in the midway position, *ardha uttan-*

asana. Therefore, the point of maximum effort, and consequently the position most difficult to stay in, is the midway position of *ardha uttanasana*.

Example 2: In the movement from uttanasana *to* samasthiti, *with the arms raised, the weight of our arms forms part of the load to be lifted, along with the weight of our trunk.* When the arms are outstretched, even though they do not weigh much, their considerable distance from the hip joints ensures that they add significantly to the effective load (torque, actually). Therefore, raising our trunk with our arms extended requires appreciably greater effort than raising our trunk with our arms folded behind our back. When our arms are folded on our back, they are much closer to the hip joints, and so their contribution to the effective load is reduced (fig. 2.37).

Example 3: Consider pascimatanasana. *The form of this asana is similar to* uttanasana, *and the final form is again maintained mainly by passive supports* (fig. 2.38). But the orientation of our body in relation to gravity has been changed. The load arm is now maximum in the final asana. Therefore, the point of maximum strain is at the start of the return movement—when we begin to lift our trunk from the bent position.

Example 4: In urdhvaprasrtapadasana, *the point of maximum effort is when we begin to lift our legs off the floor.* The hip flexors and abdominal muscles need to contract strongly to make this movement possible. The effort required decreases as we move our legs toward their final perpendicular position (fig. 2.39).

The stretching of our hamstrings increases as we near the final position.

Maintaining Balance: The Base and Center of Gravity

In any position, the weight of the body is always distributed over a certain area of the ground. This constitutes the base. The base is not limited to just the parts of the body in contact with the ground but includes the area within these points as well. Thus the size of the base is determined by how much of the body is in contact with the ground and how far apart the points of contact are. The greater the area of contact and the more spread out the points of contact, the greater the base. The base is a central factor in every asana, since it determines the stability of the position: Asanas with a larger base are more stable.

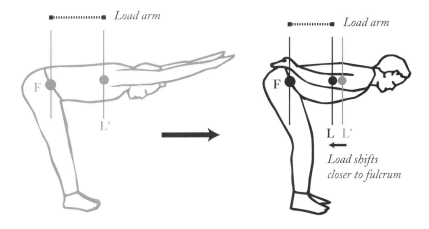

Fig. 2.37. Decrease in load arm in *ardha uttanasana* when the arms are folded on the back. In *ardha uttanasana*, the center of gravity (position of load) is at L' when the arms are extended above the head. When the arms are folded and placed on the back, the center of gravity shifts backward, closer to the hips (L). This reduces the load arm and consequently the effort required to maintain the asana.

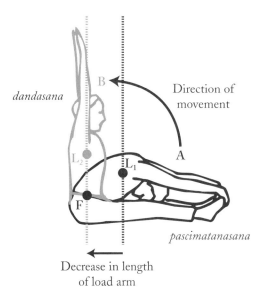

Fig. 2.38. Change in position of load and length of load arm in *pascimatanasana*. The movement is similar to that in *uttanasana*. Here too the load is the weight of the trunk, head, and arms. However, in the final asana (A), the load (L$_1$) is situated far away from the fulcrum (F). The load moves closer (L$_2$) to the fulcrum as the person returns to the initial position (B). That is, the length of the load arm is maximum in the final asana. Therefore, the effort required is also maximum at the beginning of this return movement.

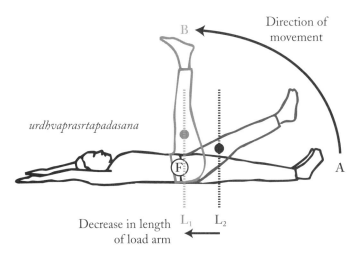

Fig. 2.39. Change in position of load and length of load arm in *urdhvaprasrtapadasana*. Here the load is the weight of the legs. In the final asana (B), the load (L$_1$) is situated very close to the fulcrum (F). The load (L$_2$) is farthest from the fulcrum in the initial stage of movement, when we begin to raise our legs off the floor (A). That is, the length of the load arm is maximum in the initial stage of the movement into the asana, and it decreases as we move further into the asana, reaching a minimum in the final position. Therefore, the effort required is also maximum at the beginning of the movement into the asana.

Let us explore the size of the base in some asanas. In standing positions, the base is the area under and between the feet (fig. 2.40). The base is smaller in *uttanasana* than in *trikonasana* and *parsva uttanasana*, in which the feet are spread apart. In seated positions, the base may or may not be larger, depending on how much of the body rests on the ground. In *padmasana*, it is much larger. In lying positions, the base is obviously very large, as a sizable section of the body is in contact with the ground.

The other factor that influences the stability of the position is the center of gravity. The center of gravity is the point through which the force of gravity apparently acts. Gravity acts as a vertical, downward force directed through the center of gravity of any object. The lower the center of gravity, the more stable the body position. Conversely, the higher the center of gravity, the more unstable the position. The center of gravity is highest in standing positions and lowest in lying positions. In general, the closer the body is to the ground, the lower the center of gravity will be.

A perpendicular line drawn from the center of gravity to the ground is called the line of gravity. The closer the line of gravity falls to the center of the base, the more stable the body position. When the line of gravity falls outside the base, the body cannot stay in balance—we tilt and fall to that side. This explains why a larger base and a lower center of gravity contribute to greater stability—in both cases, greater displacement of the body is necessary to move the line of gravity outside the base to cause destabilization.

It is important to keep in mind that the body is not a passive structure. We are used to certain positions like *samasthiti* (standing), in

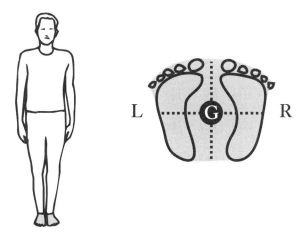

Fig. 2.40. The base in simple standing position (*samasthiti*). In general, in standing positions, the base is the area under and between the feet. Despite the small base, the position is comfortable because our body is adapted to maintain this position for extended periods.

which we are able to easily move our feet, and even hop, in any direction while maintaining our balance. In positions like *trikonasana* (in which the feet are spread laterally), the base is larger and the center of gravity is lower (fig. 2.41). But this position is not so familiar to us. The shape of the base is long from side to side and narrow from front to back. A slight forward or backward displacement of the body will place the line of gravity outside the area of the base. In contrast to *samasthiti*, in this posi-

tion it is not so easy to raise one foot and place it backward to maintain balance, and this contributes to a certain degree of instability.

But changing the shape of the base—increasing it laterally—allows us to intensify twisting and lateral-bending movements. These movements can be done with more intensity in *trikonasana* than in *samasthiti*. Because of the large side-to-side length of the base, moving the trunk to one side results in the center of gravity still falling within the

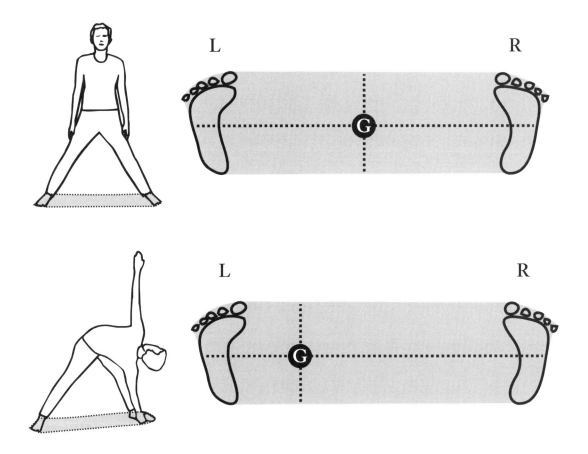

Fig. 2.41. The base in *trikonasana* is wide sideways and narrow from front to back. The line of gravity (G) falls in the center in the initial position. In the final position, it shifts to the side of the twist but still falls within the base, making the position stable.

base, thus retaining stability. Attempting a similar degree of twisting or lateral movement in *samasthiti* would result in us falling to that side. In *parsva uttanasana*, the base is not significantly different in area from that of *trikonasana*, but in shape its lateral extent is minimal, and it is extended in the forward and backward directions (fig. 2.42). Here instability can result from displacement in the lateral direction, but considerable forward or backward movement of the trunk still results in the center of gravity falling within the base. Therefore we can put much more effort into the forward-bending movements and the return movement to the upright position. These examples all show how the change in the shape and size of the base can affect the nature of movements possible in asanas.

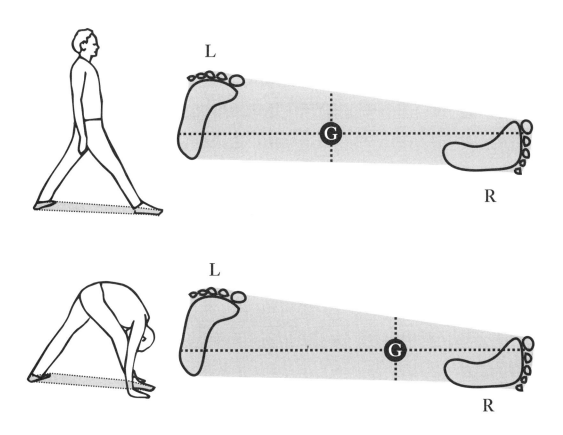

Fig. 2.42. The base in *parsva uttanasana*. In contrast to *trikonasana*, here the base is narrow sideways and long from front to back. The line of gravity (G) falls in the center in the initial position. In the final position, it shifts forward but still falls within the base, making the position stable. Because the base is narrow from side to side, it is easy to fall sideways in this asana, but we can lean forward considerably without losing balance. Therefore, we can reach forward and stretch well in this asana. This is why the forward-bending movement in this asana is very effective in stretching the back and hamstrings, even more than *uttanasana*.

Consider an asana like *ardha uttanasana*, in which the trunk is bent forward, thus moving the center of gravity forward. But the base is the same as in the standing position. Therefore, the hips move back and the body tilts backward on the feet to ensure that the center of gravity, which has shifted forward, still remains directly above the base—the feet (fig. 2.43). This is true of *uttanasana* as well, though the degree of backward tilting is less, since the trunk is closer to the legs. Very flexible people will be able to bend more completely at the hips and thus bring their trunk even closer to the legs. Therefore, they will not tilt backward as much as a stiffer person would. This point is useful in the observation and assessment of students.

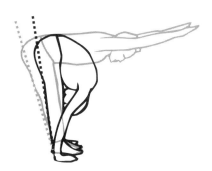

Fig. 2.43. To maintain stability, the center of gravity must always lie vertically above the base. That is, the perpendicular line drawn from the center of gravity to the ground (the line of gravity) must fall within the base. When the trunk is raised from *uttanasana* to *ardha uttanasana*, the line of gravity tends to shift forward, but the base will not change. To keep the line of gravity within the base, the body has to tilt backward.

PART TWO

Designing an Asana and Pranayama Practice

As was stated earlier, the practice of asanas must help to promote the following:

- Structural well-being, including strength, flexibility, skeletal alignment, and neuromuscular coordination
- Physiological well-being, to create optimum body function
- Psychological well-being, or clarity and balance of the mind

Of course, physical and mental well-being cannot be achieved in a single session. A gradual approach is required to lead us toward these goals. Therefore, when we design an asana practice for a particular person and a specific purpose, we need to take certain steps:

- Determine the person's starting point and the goal he or she must reach.
- Choose balanced steps leading from the starting point to the end point.
- Personalize those steps for that person.

This is the logical sequence for designing not only an asana practice but any other health program. This approach is relevant in reaching long-term goals as well as immediate objectives. We must be clear about the desired end point at all stages, in every asana, and apply the same decision-making steps. We must also continue to observe ourselves and refine our practice to maximize its effectiveness.

If you can apply this decision-making process, starting from the long-term objectives to be achieved over a period of months or years, down to each sequence of asanas, you will naturally have the ideal practice. If you continue to do this in every session, then the practice will naturally keep pace with you as you progress.

The chapters in this section follow the steps of this decision-making process. First, we discuss how to observe and assess the person to determine the starting point and end point. Next, we discuss how to formulate a sequence of balanced steps leading toward the desired goals—both short-term and long-term. That is, we explain how to use balanced, progressive sequences of asanas to lead toward a specific goal, and how progression and balance should be a part of our approach in both the short and long term. Finally, we discuss how to personalize asana movements for specific people and specific needs.

Observation and Assessment 3

I<small>T IS VERY</small> important to be aware of any imbalance in your body and breath. For example, do you have any structural imbalances? Is one of your shoulders higher than the other? Do you habitually favor one leg? Does one of your feet turn out more than the other? You can observe these features of your body with the help of a mirror or a friend. However, a comprehensive assessment of your body requires a great deal of skill and experience. With practice and with greater awareness, you will be able to observe yourself with sensitivity and accuracy. Of course, you cannot observe all aspects of your body, and you may wish to seek the help of a capable teacher.

Observation is an art that is practiced in many disciplines of life. Assessing a person in yoga is not unlike an architect assessing a construction or a doctor making a diagnosis. It requires specialized knowledge and guidance, and only some of it can be applied straight from a book. Skill will evolve with experience, but only if our methods are sound. Therefore, we do not present exhaustive lists here but a systematic approach, with examples. If you keep this approach in mind, your ability to observe and assess will improve with time, in both speed and accuracy.

WHAT TO OBSERVE AND ASSESS

The first question is, of course, what should we look for? What observations can we make that will be relevant to designing our asana practice? This is a broad question. We have to consider the structure and function of our body, the character of our breathing, and our state of mind.

We have discussed asanas, emphasizing the body primarily and the breath secondarily. But these are not the only criteria on which our practice should be based. An assessment of these alone may not always indicate what we truly need. We should also consider the condition of our mind and other areas of our life, such as our diet, habits, and personal and social interactions. It is important to keep an open mind and take all these aspects into account.

Also, structure and function are not quantities having a measurable existence separate from a person. They are meaningful only in relation to that person. Therefore, determinations concerning even simple characteristics such as strength, flexibility, or stamina depend greatly on the person's condition—age, build, weight, sex, habits, exercise tolerance, and so on—apart from such other considerations as Ayurvedic constitution. When we are assessing the breathing and other body qualities and functions, the list of associated considerations grows even longer.

It is beyond the scope of this book to attempt to list everything that should be observed, especially in yoga therapy, where the list can grow very long. This chapter concerns the assessment of the structural characteristics of the body and the qualities of the breath.

Observing the Breath

Movement and breathing always go together in asanas. To assess the quality of the movement, you must observe the breath as well. The character of your breath indicates the ease with which you are doing the movement. The rate and depth of your breathing are general indicators of the level of exertion to which you are being subjected. A person with greater stamina and cardiovascular fitness will have less shortness of breath on similar exertion. Therefore, to decide whether you should increase or decrease the effort involved in your practice, it is necessary to observe your breath.

It is important to observe your breath before the practice of asanas is started and during the three phases in any asana: the movement into the asana, the stay in the asana, and the movement out of the asana. Each of these can provide valuable insight. The following are useful points to observe:

- Do you emphasize chest breathing or abdominal breathing?
- What does your breath sound like?
- How would you describe the quality of your breath before your practice, while resting, and between asanas?
- How would you describe the quality of your breath when you stay in asanas?

The most important point concerning breathing in asanas is that your breath should be long and smooth. If it is not, you must determine the cause of the disturbance and restructure the movements and breathing to restore the length and smoothness of your breath. Disturbed breathing detracts from the central goal of asana practice, which is a state of balance. This is probably the most important reason observing your breath is of vital importance in the practice of asanas.

Observing Body Structure and Alignment

Learning how to observe body structure and alignment is especially important for yoga teachers. If you are a yoga student, you can also use this information to develop your own awareness and to ensure that your yoga

teacher is giving you an appropriate practice.

For example, you may be able to get into the asana called *utkatasana*. However, in order to do this asana properly, you need a strong back, flexible ankles and hips, and strong legs and knees. Therefore, it is important for you to assess whether you can comfortably do the asanas that prepare your body for *utkatasana*: *salabhasana, vajrasana,* and *ardha utkatasana* (fig. 3.1).

Several important aspects of people's body structure can be observed when they are in normal relaxed positions—as they walk into a room or in the standing, seated, or lying positions:

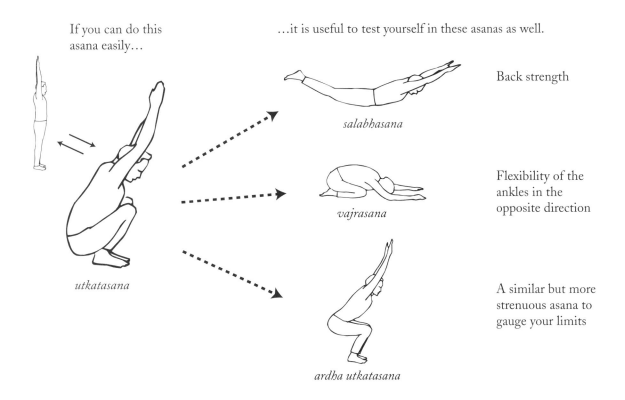

If you can do this asana easily…

…it is useful to test yourself in these asanas as well.

salabhasana

Back strength

vajrasana

Flexibility of the ankles in the opposite direction

utkatasana

ardha utkatasana

A similar but more strenuous asana to gauge your limits

Fig. 3.1. An example of correlating multiple observations: *utkatasana.*

- Their height, weight, and build. Are they heavily built or lightly built? Compact or flabby? Muscular, overweight, or thin?
- Their age, not just chronologically but physiologically as well.

Ask about any important health conditions they may have. Next, observe the alignment of the various body areas. The deviation may be along any one of the three axes. The exact possibilities depend on the region (fig. 3.2):

- Head and neck
  — Rotation or slanting of the head to either side
  — Elevation or depression of the head
  — Forward deviation of the head
- Shoulders
  — Level of the shoulders—are they in line with each other, or is one shoulder depressed or elevated?
  — Rounding of the shoulders, commonly associated with an increase in the thoracic curvature
- Spine
  Observe the spine and its curvatures, as indicated by the shape of the back:
  — Cervical: The position of the head in the relaxed state is a good indicator of changes in this curvature.

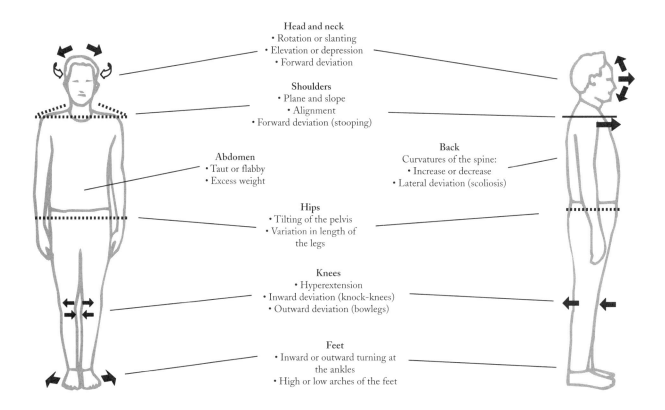

Fig. 3.2. Observe general body structure and structural misalignment before commencing the design of an asana program.

—Thoracic: Look for increase in the thoracic curvature (kyphosis). This may be reflected in rounded shoulders and a stooping appearance.

—Lumbar: Look for an increase in the lumbar curvature (lordosis). Remember that this can be associated with a forward rotation of the pelvis.

—Check for any lateral deviation (scoliosis) of the spine.

• Hips

—Is the pelvis tilted forward or backward? The forward and backward tilting of the pelvis can generally be assessed from the shape of the back and the posture.

—Is one hip higher than the other?

—Are the legs equal in length?

This may be difficult to assess, especially in the standing position. It is usually most easily seen in inverted asanas, but inversion is not for everyone. Therefore, observation in more than one body position may be needed.

• Knees

—Are the knees hyperextended?

—Are they deviated laterally either inward (knock-knees) or outward (bowlegs)?

• Feet

—Is either foot or both turned outward or inward? Such deviations of one foot are common as a consequence of injury.

—Observe the arches. Are the feet flat?

Most of us have some uneven development of the two sides of our body. The fact that we are either right- or left-handed by preference

is enough to ensure this. The degree of the discrepancy determines how much we need to account for it when designing the practice.

Figure 3.3 gives examples of movements that can be useful in working with some of the misalignments listed above.

Assessing Strength and Flexibility

In designing an asana practice, we usually do not try to assess the strength or flexibility at each joint. Instead, we generally take advantage of the composite nature of the movements in asanas to assemble an overall picture of our strength and flexibility. We may sometimes check a particular joint or body part in therapeutic settings. Remember that strength is the force with which we can do a movement, and flexibility can be judged by the range of motion possible at a joint. Strength and flexibility together determine the force and range of a movement.

Flexibility can always be a limiting factor, even in movements that require strength. Movements that are assisted by gravity are not the only tests of flexibility. Even movements that require considerable effort or strength may be limited by the inability of complementary body parts to stretch. Raising our legs from the lying position while keeping them straight is an example of this. Not only does this movement require considerable strength, it also requires the hamstrings to stretch (fig. 3.4). If you have adequate strength but inflexible hamstrings, you will not be able to keep your legs straight. So this movement also helps you to assess your hip

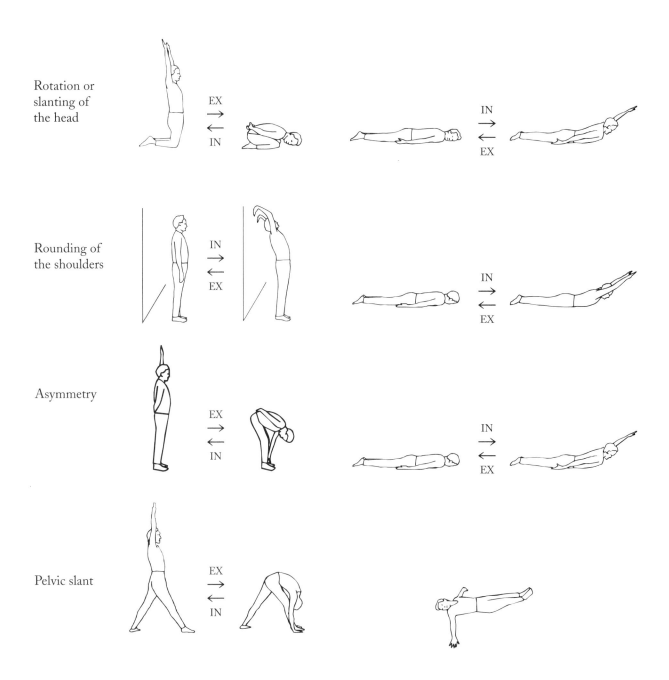

Rotation or slanting of the head

Rounding of the shoulders

Asymmetry

Pelvic slant

Fig. 3.3. Examples of asanas that can be useful in working with structural misalignments.

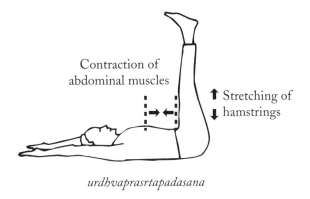

urdhvaprasrtapadasana

Fig. 3.4. Both strength and flexibility are required to move into or stay in *urdhvaprasrtapadasana*.

flexibility as well as the ability of the hamstrings to stretch.

We usually do not test strength against resistance in asanas; the weight of the body is used as the load. Therefore, in asanas, we use movements that resist gravity to check for a lack of strength.

The inability to do a movement may be due to both weakness and stiffness in an elderly person, but it is less likely to be due to weakness in an otherwise normal younger adult. For example, a forty-five-year old man who is unable to raise his left arm fully but is otherwise normal is probably stiff and not weak. His stiffness could be due simply to a lack of use or perhaps to some underlying pathological process. But a sixty-five-year-old woman who is unable to do *salabhasana* well could certainly be weak as well as stiff. Men,

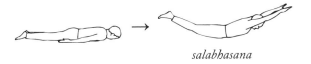

salabhasana

who are generally more muscular than women, tend to develop similar levels of flexibility only with greater effort than women. The person's weight and build must also be taken into account.

HOW TO OBSERVE AND ASSESS

Making the Assessment Personal

You can assess your strength and flexibility during movements into and out of asanas and also during the stay in asanas.

In your assessment, you should choose movements with a level of intensity that is appropriate for you. Depending on your assessment of your general characteristics, you should decide on a particular grade of difficulty and test how comfortable you are with it. If you are comfortable with simple movements, you can progress to those with greater intensity. Figure 3.5 illustrates the examples discussed below.

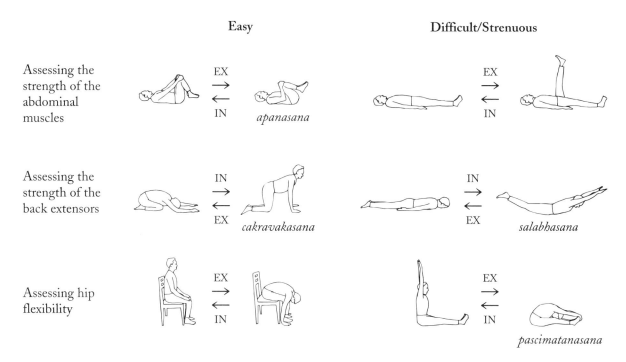

Fig. 3.5. Personalizing the assessment process: examples of easy and strenuous movements to test the strength or flexibility of various body areas.

For example, you may want to assess the strength of your abdominal muscles. The movement you select will depend on your age and strength. If you are an elderly man, you could try *apanasana*, but if you are a fit young woman, you could raise one leg straight off the floor.

Similarly, you can use a range of movements to test the strength of your back extensors. Here too you must select an asana that is appropriate for you. For example, the elderly man might do *cakravakasana*, while the fit young woman could try *salabhasana*. The same concept applies to the assessment of flexibility. Hip flexibility, for example, can be assessed in movements ranging from

bending down while seated on a chair to *pascimatanasana*.

It goes without saying that, like strength and flexibility, asymmetry or misalignment must also be assessed in movements appropriate for you. This can be done by moving the limbs individually in asymmetrical asanas and comparing the movement on the two sides or by observing the difference between the two sides in symmetrical asanas. Two such common observations are the out-

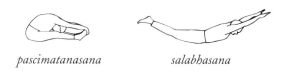

pascimatanasana   *salabhasana*

ward deviation of either leg in *salabhasana* or the outward rotation of one of the feet in *pascimatanasana*.

Making Multiple Observations in One Asana

As asanas are composite movements, several observations can be made in each asana. In any particular asana, the work is concentrated more at certain regions of your body, making it easy to observe the characteristics of body structure in those regions as you do that asana. As your experience increases, the number of points you can observe in each asana will increase, and you will also be able to observe your breathing at the same time. Consider *cakravakasana,* for instance (fig. 3.6). In this asana, the back is supported by all four limbs. The natural shape of the back in this asana is a useful indicator of the extent of the curvatures of the spine. Accentuation of the lower back curvature is usually evident in this position. The position of the head gives a clue to the curvature of the neck. In the final position, this asana allows gentle flexion and extension of your back. The hips can be kept relatively immobile, and the movements of the back can be observed fairly exclusively. While the back is quite comfortably supported, the neck muscles have to support the weight of the head. The strain on the neck muscles is greater than in the upright position. Therefore your ability to raise your head in this position will reveal any weakness of your neck muscles. Note, however, that a lack of flexibility could also be the cause for the limited movement of the head. You should try moving your neck in other positions to determine whether your neck is weak or stiff.

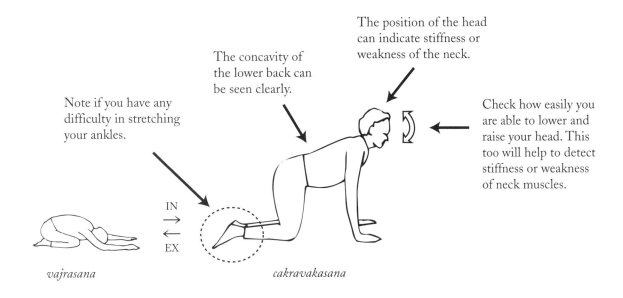

The position of the head can indicate stiffness or weakness of the neck.

The concavity of the lower back can be seen clearly.

Note if you have any difficulty in stretching your ankles.

Check how easily you are able to lower and raise your head. This too will help to detect stiffness or weakness of neck muscles.

IN
EX

vajrasana   *cakravakasana*

Fig. 3.6. Multiple observations in one asana: *cakravakasana.*

In *cakravakasana*, you can also assess the flexibility of your ankles (which are plantar flexed in this position). You can also assess the flexibility of your hips in this asana, because in the starting position (*vajrasana*) the hips are completely flexed, with the trunk bent over the thighs. However, if you are overweight or stiff, you may have difficulty in bending fully in *vajrasana*.

Keep in mind that while the primary movement in an asana may involve one muscle group, others have to contract to keep the rest of the body stable. It is important to observe these groups of muscles as well. Take, for example, leg lifting in the lying position (*urdhvaprasrtapadasana*). In this movement, the role of the abdominal muscles is to stabilize the pelvis so that the hip flexors can act from there to raise the legs. In this asana, therefore, you need to observe not only your thighs and abdominal muscles but your back and neck as well (fig. 3.7). If your neck arches and lifts off the floor, it could mean that you lack adequate strength in those muscle groups that support

the movement, even though the actual movement is occurring in a different part of your body. This is important, because care needs to be devoted to adequately preparing all areas of your body. For example, before attempting a shoulder stand, you must be able to do *urdhvaprasrtapadasana* and ensure that you have adequate strength in the neck and the back to lift your legs safely and then to maintain your torso and legs in an inverted position.

Correlating Multiple Observations

Single observations have limited value. We cannot reach a conclusion based on observations made in just one asana or only one movement. There can be many causes for restricted or unusual body movements. It is important to cross-check and confirm our conclusions by assessing ourselves in other movements and positions.

Consider *utkatasana*. The final position places stress on the ankles and knees and demands flexibility in these areas as well as in

It is important to observe the neck and upper body as well.

The movement primarily involves this part of the body.

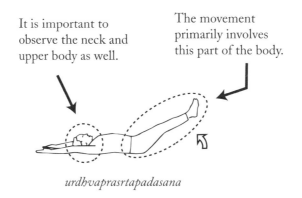

urdhvaprasrtapadasana

Fig. 3.7. It is important to observe body regions other than the primary ones (where the movement takes place).

the hips. The return movement requires strength in the back. If you are used to similar positions such as sitting on the floor, you may be able to do this asana very comfortably. However, you may be able to do *utkatasana* easily simply because you have flat feet. You should observe yourself in other asanas to see whether you have strength and flexibility in the parts of your body that are involved in doing *utkatasana* (see fig. 3.1 on p. 65). For example, you could use *salabhasana* as a test for strength in your back, *vajrasana* to test the range of movement in your ankles in the opposite direction (dorsiflexion), and *ardha utkatasana*, a more strenuous asana, to give you an idea of your limits.

It is also important to observe whether you are doing the asana or movement in the correct manner. It is not enough just to be able to do it; you must have the required structural and functional attributes (strength, flexibility, and alignment) that will enable you to do the movement without strain. If you do not have these attributes, you may be able to make the movement or get into the position depicted for an asana, but you will be forcing your body into the position and holding it using inappropriate muscle work and alignment. This is of no help in improving your body structure or function. Therefore, it is important to note the ease with which you are able to do the movements and breathing involved in asana practice. The quality of your breathing is the key to this assessment.

WHEN TO OBSERVE AND ASSESS

Observing yourself and refining your conclusions must go on throughout your practice. That is, you must observe and assess yourself continuously:

- Before doing an asana
- As you move into the asana (fig. 3.8)
- While you stay in the asana (fig. 3.9)

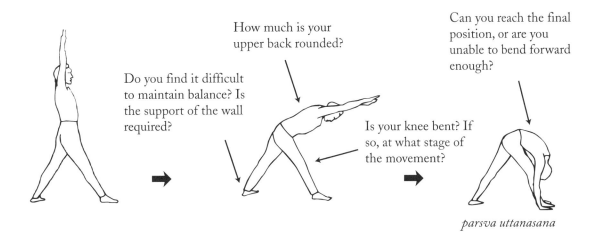

How much is your upper back rounded?

Do you find it difficult to maintain balance? Is the support of the wall required?

Can you reach the final position, or are you unable to bend forward enough?

Is your knee bent? If so, at what stage of the movement?

parsva uttanasana

Fig. 3.8. Observation during movement into *parsva uttanasana*.

- As you move out of the asana (fig. 3.10)
- After doing the asana

Each phase offers you an opportunity to observe various characteristics of your body and breath. Which part of the body you observe and which characteristics you seek to assess will depend on the asana used. Figure 3.11 illustrates how observations can be made in all phases in one asana.

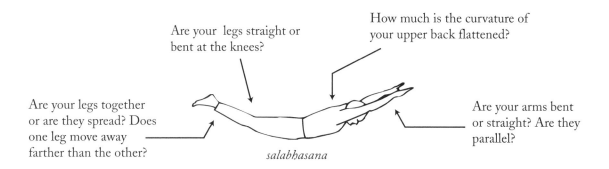

Are your legs straight or bent at the knees?

How much is the curvature of your upper back flattened?

Are your legs together or are they spread? Does one leg move away farther than the other?

Are your arms bent or straight? Are they parallel?

salabhasana

Fig. 3.9. Observation during the stay in *salabhasana*.

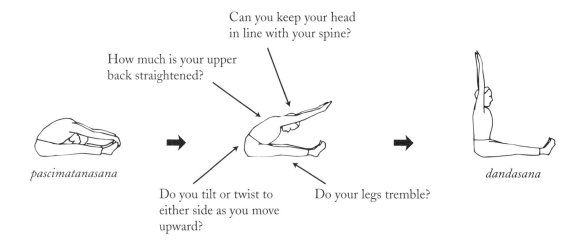

Can you keep your head in line with your spine?

How much is your upper back straightened?

pascimatanasana

Do you tilt or twist to either side as you move upward?

Do your legs tremble?

dandasana

Fig. 3.10. Observation during movement out of *pascimatanasana*.

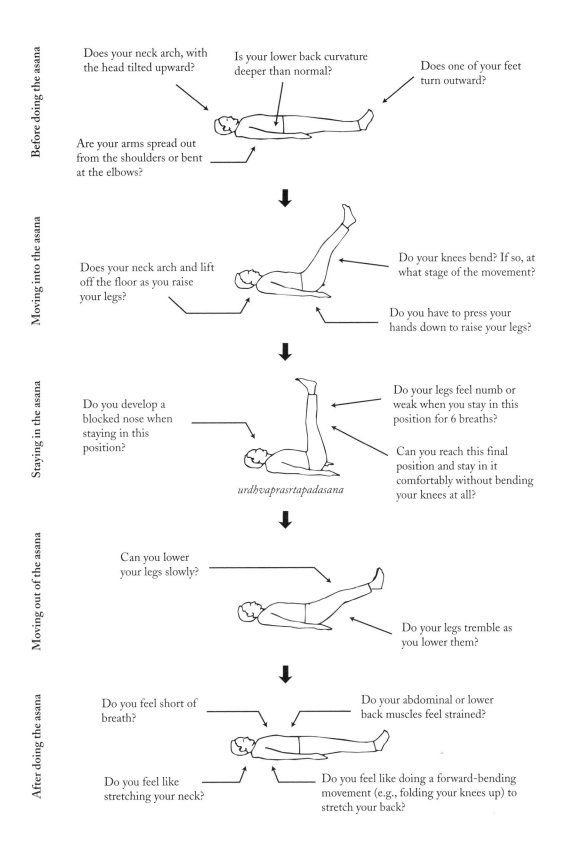

Before doing the asana

Does your neck arch, with the head tilted upward?

Is your lower back curvature deeper than normal?

Does one of your feet turn outward?

Are your arms spread out from the shoulders or bent at the elbows?

Moving into the asana

Does your neck arch and lift off the floor as you raise your legs?

Do your knees bend? If so, at what stage of the movement?

Do you have to press your hands down to raise your legs?

Staying in the asana

Do you develop a blocked nose when staying in this position?

Do your legs feel numb or weak when you stay in this position for 6 breaths?

Can you reach this final position and stay in it comfortably without bending your knees at all?

urdhvaprasrtapadasana

Moving out of the asana

Can you lower your legs slowly?

Do your legs tremble as you lower them?

After doing the asana

Do you feel short of breath?

Do your abdominal or lower back muscles feel strained?

Do you feel like stretching your neck?

Do you feel like doing a forward-bending movement (e.g., folding your knees up) to stretch your back?

Fig. 3.11. Observation in all five phases of *urdhvaprasrtapadasana*.

Sequencing: Progression with Balance

4

THE GOAL of asana practice is to maintain or restore health in body and mind. Much confusion in the field of yoga arises from considering the form of an asana to be the goal—to be an end in itself. This belief is usually based on the assumption that a particular body position confers some mystical or occult benefits. This assumption in turn stems from a literal interpretation of ancient yoga texts, many of which describe the final form of various asanas and the benefits they confer. The cause-effect relationship between the asana and the benefit, and the nature of the benefit itself, are not defined in terms of modern medical science in the ancient yoga texts. The descriptions in the texts on yoga are based on Ayurveda and use concepts more specific to yoga, like prana, *apana*, *nadis,* and kundalini. Some of these concepts are dis-cussed in later chapters. However, you must be aware that forcing yourself to "perform" asanas and taking literally the recommendations from ancient texts may not result in good health.

For example, consider *pascimatanasana,* a seated asana in which the upper half of the body is bent forward over the lower half. The main requirement for assuming such a position is adequate flexibility at the hip joints and the ability of the hamstrings to stretch. The strength of the back and other muscles is of little importance. It is possible to assume the ideal form of *pascimatanasana* very easily without developing adequate strength in the back. In fact, many fit people can do this asana simply as a result of practicing similar movements over a period of time.

There is nothing wrong in being able to

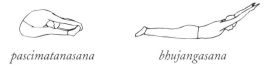

pascimatanasana   *bhujangasana*

do this asana well. It indicates that the person is very flexible. The question, however, is whether someone has both strength and flexibility. Can he or she do opposing movements like *bhujangasana* with equal ease? The flexibility at the hips must be accompanied by corresponding strength in the back. If not, the practice is fostering imbalance in the body. Further, it is important not to exceed our limits: Flexibility is good, but hyperflexibility is not.

In summary, assuming the final form of the asana is not the purpose of our practice. The benefits that we derive from the movements and breathing are. When we understand the movement and breathing involved in an asana, we have understood the asana. There are practically innumerable ways of combining movement and breathing so as to have a particular effect. That is, with any one purpose in mind, it is possible to suggest a variety of movement/breathing combinations that will produce the required effect. In addition, the intensity of the movements can range from extremely gentle to exceedingly strong.

As our goal is the optimal functioning of the body and the mind, our approach must be comprehensive, balanced, clear, and flexible. It must pay attention to several important factors, including the following:

• Our condition and needs. Are we stiff or flexible, strong or weak? In which parts of our body? Which movements should we concentrate on?
• Any illness or imbalances in our body
• The use of our breath to develop stamina
• What we have done before our practice and what we will do after our practice

We must consider all of these issues if we are to use asanas to work effectively toward a specific purpose.

Arranging asanas for a particular purpose for a particular person is both a science and an art. In this chapter, we discuss the science of designing a sequence of movements and breathing to attain a particular purpose. We are assuming that the student has a normal degree of fitness.

In assembling a sequence of asanas, we seek to establish a progression of movements that will lead to the development of the characteristics that we seek. We should always start with simple movements and gradually progress to the more demanding ones. The starting point for each person should be clear from observing and assessing his or her current state. Forcing the body into positions to which it is unaccustomed is of no benefit. It also carries a significant risk of injury and is of course completely contrary to the spirit of yoga.

We must have a clear understanding of the effects of the movements involved in getting into, staying in, and getting out of each asana. When we describe a movement as difficult or easy, we are judging the intensity of the work involved in making that movement. This presumes that we understand which part of the

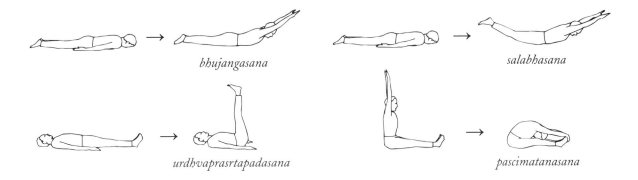

bhujangasana

salabhasana

urdhvaprasrtapadasana

pascimatanasana

body is being worked on by the movement and in what way.

For example, *bhujangasana* and *salabhasana* require strong contraction of the muscles of the back; *urdhvaprasrtapadasana* involves powerful contraction of the abdominal muscles; and *pascimatanasana* requires considerable stretching of the hamstrings and flexibility at the hips. It is evident that in order to design a sequence that will prepare the body to do one of these asanas, we must select a progression of movements that gradually increases the work on those parts of the body. This will lead to the development of the structural qualities that are necessary to assume that asana.

It cannot be overemphasized that structural, physiological, and psychological well-being are the true indicators of progress; the mere performance of asanas is not. For example, our aim should be to develop strength in the back muscles and not simply to do *salabhasana*. Indeed, whether we use *salabhasana* for this purpose is irrelevant.

It is obvious that health and well-being cannot be enhanced by practicing only one or two asanas. We need to practice a variety of asanas. But how do we choose which asanas to do? In what order should we do them? In this chapter, we discuss how to choose appropriate asanas and how to arrange them in order.

GENERAL GUIDELINES FOR EFFECTIVE SEQUENCING

A sequence is a series of steps leading to a particular goal. First, it is important to be clear of the goal—the attributes you need to develop. Before you can design a sequence of asanas, you need to know where you are starting from and where you are going. Movement toward your goal is progress. Therefore, progress is defined by your needs. To design an effective sequence of asanas, you must be clear about your starting point and realistic in your goals.

All of us possess the structural, functional, and psychological qualities of health to varying degrees. But most of us are lacking in one or more of these qualities. Building the attributes of health that we lack—structural, functional, or psychological—should be the goal of a sequence of asanas. Building strength could be the goal for one person. Increasing flexibility could be the goal for someone else. For another person, the goal might be to resolve a structural disorder.

Therefore, begin by assessing yourself. Be clear about which characteristics you need to develop and maintain in your body and mind. Do you lack strength or flexibility or both? Do you have any structural imbalances in your body that you should work toward correcting or at least refrain from aggravating? Do you need to work toward improving the inhalation or the exhalation? If you have a specific illness, your goals may be clear. Otherwise, to answer these questions, you will need to observe and assess yourself before you start.

Having identified your goals, look for progress. Sequencing involves placing asanas in order in a session and also over several sessions. We need to know how to place asanas in a balanced, progressive order in a single sequence. We also need to know how to design a series of balanced, progressive sequences over a period of time, usually several months.

Planning Sequences over Time

Strength, flexibility, alignment, and good breathing cannot be forced on the body. They must be developed gradually and intelligently over time. If you have back pain, for example, you may need to develop flexibility in your back. Your long-term goal might be to do *pascimatanasana*. Forcing yourself into that position right away would only worsen your back pain. You need to develop flexibility gradually. To do that, you need to know the

pascimatanasana

key movements and breathing to incorporate in several sequences over some months, so that you can gradually stretch your back muscles (fig. 4.1).

Though a sequence of asanas may be primarily designed to develop one aspect of body structure or breathing, it must avoid creating imbalance in other areas. For example, if you have excessively flexible hips, increasing your flexibility further is pointless. Developing strength may be the most important goal of your asana practice. But, while building strength, you must take care not to aggravate any existing structural misalignment, disturb the quality of your breathing, or create functional disorders.

Improper sequences of asanas will create an imbalance between strength and flexibility. Building strength and flexibility usually requires movements that are opposite in direction. Therefore, it is easy to sacrifice one when working toward the other. Structural misalignment is often a consequence of such imbalance. In most people, either strength or flexibility will need to be emphasized. However, as you develop one of these qualities, make sure that you also maintain the other.

Designing Each Sequence

Progress in asanas is made in small steps. Once you are clear about the key steps on your path, design each sequence of asanas to

Forward-bending movements

Backward-bending movements

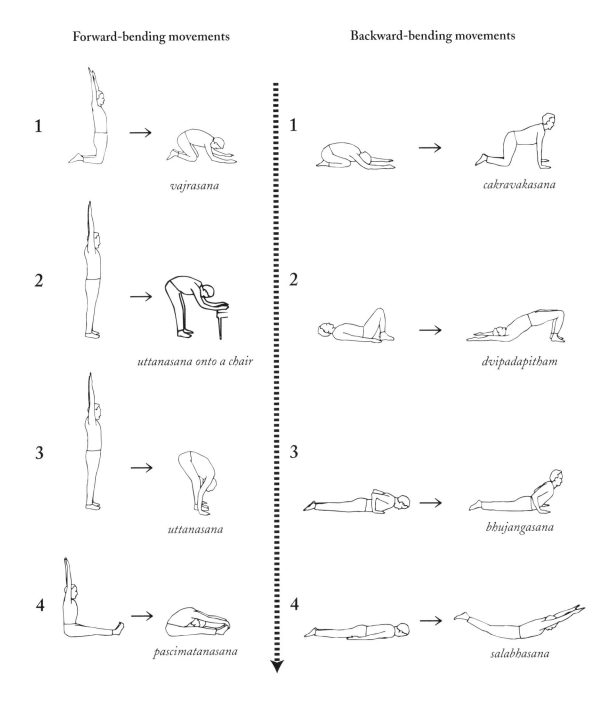

1 → *vajrasana*

1 → *cakravakasana*

2 → *uttanasana onto a chair*

2 → *dvipadapitham*

3 → *uttanasana*

3 → *bhujangasana*

4 → *pascimatanasana*

4 → *salabhasana*

Fig. 4.1. Progression of forward-bending and backward-bending movements.

lead you from where you are to the next point on the path. For example, if you are in bed with severe back pain, design your first sequence to decrease your pain. In the next sequence, you should probably try to progress to sitting on the bed. The next sequence may consist of simple movements from the seated position designed to increase your mobility. You may have to practice each sequence for a week or more before you are ready to move on to the next one. It depends on your condition and your goal.

Within each sequence of asanas there should be a logical progression, just as in any other exercise program. Start with preparation or warming up. Then incorporate the key elements in your sequence. This should be the most demanding phase of your practice. Then follow this with some movements or breathing to relieve any stress that may have been created.

To avoid creating imbalance, always relieve the stress created by the more intense asanas in the sequence. This is essential for deriving maximal benefit from the asanas that follow. It not only helps to avoid creating imbalance but also helps maximize progress. Use gentle backward-bending movements to relieve any stress from intense forward-bending movements. Use gentle forward-bending movements to balance the effect of intense backward, twisting, and lateral movements.

Asymmetrical movements will help maintain structural alignment. Twisting movements are especially useful. This may not be possible in some therapeutic applications, but it is very important in sequences for a fit person.

Assessment and sequencing should be done continuously. Progress and change are continuous processes. Therefore, there is always room to modify any sequence of asanas based on your assessment of your body, breathing, and mind that day. You may choose to rearrange the asanas you do, or change some of them to maximize the benefit of that practice session. This is a skill that comes with practice.

INEFFECTIVE APPROACHES TO SEQUENCING

Doing Asanas in a Random Order

We could choose some asanas that we like or are comfortable in and practice them in no particular order. For example, we could simply do whichever asanas we feel like doing that day. The problem with this approach is the lack of a clear goal. We cannot be sure of the result of our practice if we place our asanas in a random sequence. In fact, random sequencing is actually no sequencing, because it does not have a clear purpose. Since asanas are done one after another, each asana works on a body that has been affected by the previous asana. As we already explained, we must relax the areas that have been stressed by one asana before moving to the next. For example, doing a twisting movement after staying in an intense backward-bending asana is not a good idea. The muscles that were strongly contracted during the backward-bending asana should first be stretched slowly and relaxed, usually by a gentle forward-bending movement, before the twisting movement is attempted. Randomly ordering asanas does not take such interactions into account.

In short, this approach does not incorporate any logical progression, and it can also lead to imbalance.

Doing Similar Asanas Together in One Sequence

We can group asanas together based on their similar direction of movement or body position. On this basis, we can do similar asanas in a sequence. Some examples could be: a session of all forward-bending asanas, or all backward-bending asanas, or all standing asanas. In these practices, we can certainly incorporate a logical progression—from simple to difficult asanas over a period of time, and within each sequence—but they are defective because they are not balanced.

If you do only forward-bending movements, over time you will develop flexibility and long exhalation but not strength or inhalation. Conversely, if you do only backward-bending movements, you will develop strength and inhalation at the expense of flexibility and exhalation. Using only one body position in a practice is not a good idea because it will place prolonged or disproportionate stress on some muscle groups while ignoring others.

This approach can incorporate a logical progression, but it will create imbalance.

EXAMPLES OF SEQUENCING

Three Sequences for Increasing Back Strength

The following sequences are designed for a fit person. The goal is to increase the strength of the back muscles. This practice should not be used in therapy for conditions involving back pain.

The key asanas that we work toward in these three sequences are shown in order of increasing intensity in figure 4.2. They consist of backward-bending movements mainly from the lying position. Each succeeding asana requires greater strength in the back. These movements are gradually introduced in the practice over the three sequences (fig. 4.3).

In the same three sequences, you can also see another series of movements that help increase back strength (figs. 4.4, 4.5). These standing backward-bending movements always precede the backward-bending movements done from a lying position. This is because they are easier than the lying backward-bending movements and serve to prepare the body for them.

Within each sequence, there is a phase of preparation or warming up, consisting of mild to moderate forward- and backward-bending movements from the standing and kneeling positions. There is free movement in all these asanas. The most intense asanas in the practice, the backward-bending movements done from a lying position, are always introduced only after these preparatory asanas.

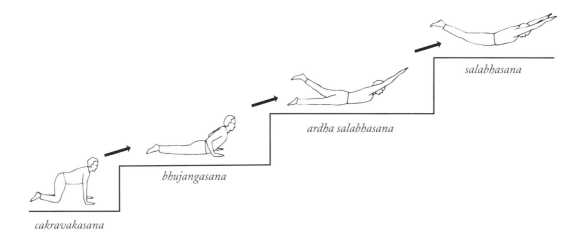

Fig. 4.2. Progression of lying backward-bending movements for increasing back strength.

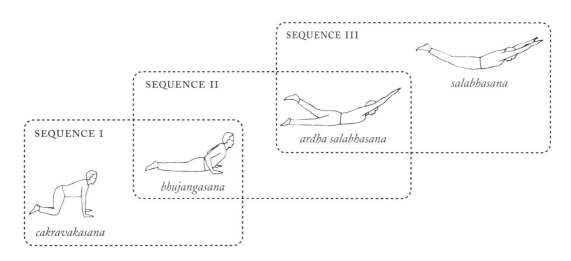

Fig. 4.3. Distribution of the lying backward-bending asanas over the three sequences.

To create balance in each sequence, all intense movements are followed by either a short rest in the lying position or by a gentle movement in an opposite direction. Because these sequences are aimed at developing back strength, all the intense movements in them are backward-bending movements. All of these back bends are followed by rest, by simple forward-bending movements, or by both.

All three sequences end with a seated forward-bending movement and a seated rest, leaving the person ready to do pranayama.

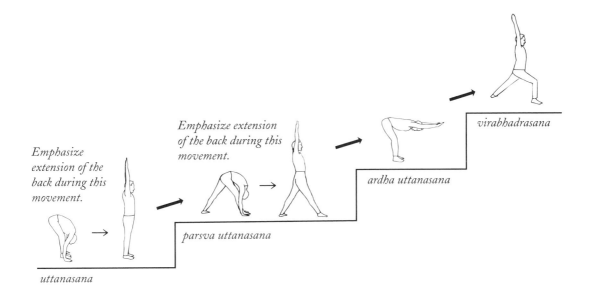

Fig. 4.4. Progression of standing asanas for increasing back strength.

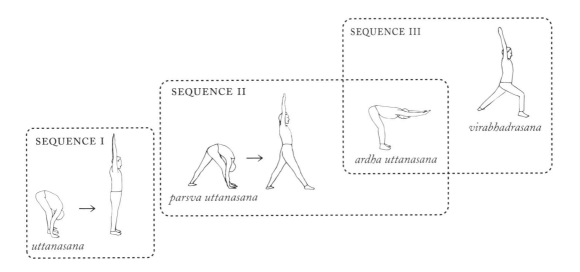

Fig. 4.5. Distribution of the standing asanas over the three sequences.

Sequencing for Strength: Sequence I

The **compensatory movements** at several stages in the sequence are illustrated here as shown below.

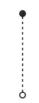

Relatively intense asana.

Asanas to relieve areas stressed by the intense asana and avoid imbalance.

Note that there are **asymmetrical movements** in this sequence, marked .

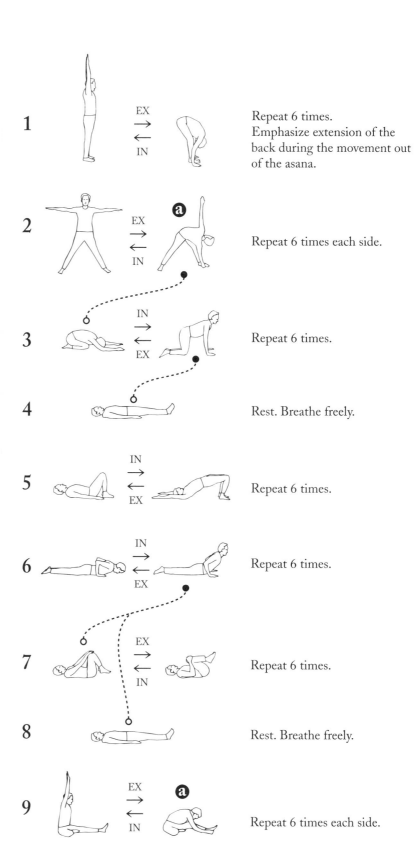

1   EX → ← IN
Repeat 6 times.
Emphasize extension of the back during the movement out of the asana.

2   EX → ← IN   **a**
Repeat 6 times each side.

3   IN → ← EX
Repeat 6 times.

4
Rest. Breathe freely.

5   IN → ← EX
Repeat 6 times.

6   IN → ← EX
Repeat 6 times.

7   EX → ← IN
Repeat 6 times.

8
Rest. Breathe freely.

9   EX → ← IN   **a**
Repeat 6 times each side.

10
Rest.

Sequencing for Strength: Sequence II

The **compensatory movements** and asymmetrical movements are illustrated as in sequence I.

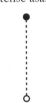

Relatively intense asana.

Asanas to relieve areas stressed by the intense asana and avoid imbalance.

Note that there are **asymmetrical movements** in this sequence, marked **ⓐ** .

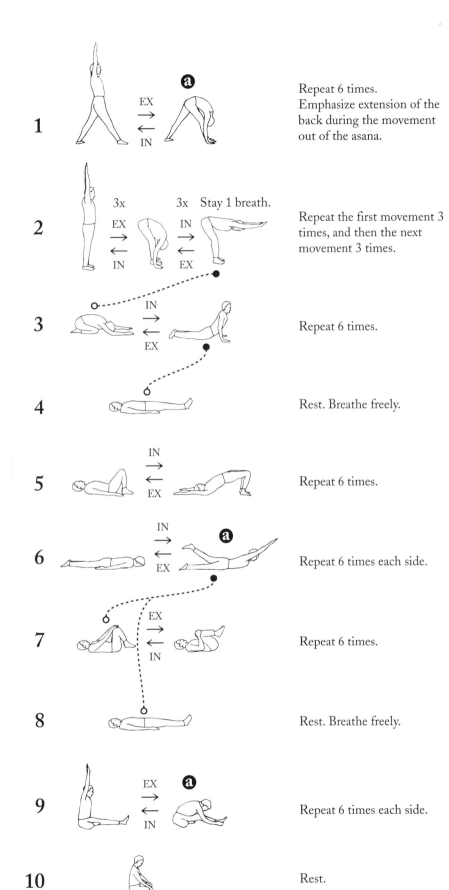

1 — EX → ← IN — ⓐ — Repeat 6 times. Emphasize extension of the back during the movement out of the asana.

2 — 3x EX → ← IN — 3x IN → ← EX — Stay 1 breath. — Repeat the first movement 3 times, and then the next movement 3 times.

3 — IN → ← EX — Repeat 6 times.

4 — Rest. Breathe freely.

5 — IN → ← EX — Repeat 6 times.

6 — IN → ← EX — ⓐ — Repeat 6 times each side.

7 — EX → ← IN — Repeat 6 times.

8 — Rest. Breathe freely.

9 — EX → ← IN — ⓐ — Repeat 6 times each side.

10 — Rest.

Sequencing for Strength: Sequence III

The **compensatory movements** and asymmetrical movements are illustrated as in sequence II.

Relatively intense asana.

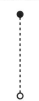

Asanas to relieve areas stressed by the intense asana and avoid imbalance.

Note that there are **asymmetrical movements** in this sequence, marked **ⓐ** .

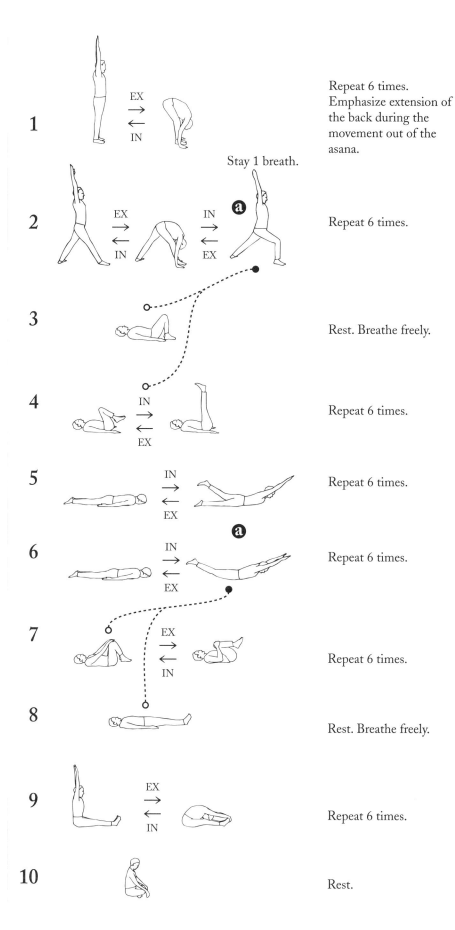

1 — EX → / IN ← — Repeat 6 times. Emphasize extension of the back during the movement out of the asana.

Stay 1 breath.

2 — EX → / IN ← — IN → / EX ← — **ⓐ** Repeat 6 times.

3 — Rest. Breathe freely.

4 — IN → / EX — Repeat 6 times.

5 — IN → / EX ← — Repeat 6 times.

ⓐ

6 — IN → / EX ← — Repeat 6 times.

7 — EX → / IN ← — Repeat 6 times.

8 — Rest. Breathe freely.

9 — EX → / IN ← — Repeat 6 times.

10 — Rest.

Preparatory Sequences

Below are three examples of how to prepare for an asana. These examples present only the general concepts based on movements and breathing that are applicable to everyone. In reality, however, an assessment of your special needs is essential before you attempt any one of these asanas.

As we have said, the goal of the practice is to develop the degree of fitness that will enable us to do the asana properly. This leads to the question, What does it mean to do the asana "properly"? The answer lies in the character of our breathing while we do the asana. If we force ourselves into an asana without adequate preparation and stay there by sheer effort, our breathing will be disturbed. Therefore, to do an asana as it should be done, we must be able to stay in that asana and breathe steadily and comfortably, generally for about six breaths.

Doing an asana in any other way can lead to imbalance. Patience is necessary. Preparation will take time. In the case of asanas like *dhanurasana, dvipada viparitakarani, uttana mayurasana,* and *urdhva dhanurasana,* preparing the body and breath may take several months, even for a fit person. A person who is unwell should not be doing these asanas at all.

Preparation for dhanurasana. We will now discuss preparatory and balancing movements for *dhanurasana,* also known as the bow pose.

The first step in designing a sequence leading to an asana is to understand the work

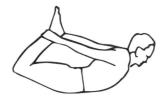

dhanurasana

or effort involved in it—what are the areas of stress? These are the areas that require careful attention and maximum preparation.

An analysis of *dhanurasana* will reveal the following:

- The arms are extended backward and the shoulders are pulled back.
- The curvature of the upper back is decreased and those of the lower back and neck are increased. This effect on the curvatures of the spine is pronounced. It is brought about by both the contraction of the muscles of the back and the drawing-back of the shoulders.
- The thigh muscles are strongly contracted and the knees are under considerable stress. The contraction of the thigh muscles tries to straighten the knees, but they are prevented from moving and held in the half-folded position by the hands. For this reason, the arms and shoulders are also subjected to the same force—the backward pull on them is significant.
- The entire front of the body (chest, abdomen, thighs) is stretched, with the abdomen resting on the floor.

Some useful movements to prepare the body for this asana are given in figure 4.6.

Knees and thigh muscles   **Abdomen and chest**

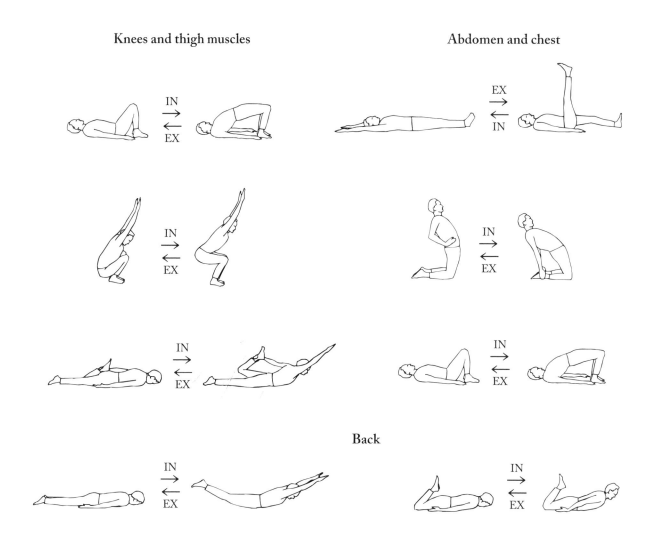

Back

Fig. 4.6. Asanas to prepare different areas of the body to do *dhanurasana*.

Note that this classification is only an outline. Each asana works on several areas of the body, and we often incorporate many significant alterations into a practice. When we design a sequence, we consider more than one area of work and more than one effect of an asana. Furthermore, we also take into account the interactions of these effects, as the asanas done in a single session follow each other in a short span of time. This leads to an overlap of their effects.

Naturally, the sequence is not ideal for everyone. We all have areas of strength and weakness, and these will determine our choice of asanas. Different preparatory movements will be more appropriate for different persons, depending on which areas need more attention.

Sequence for *Dhanurasana*

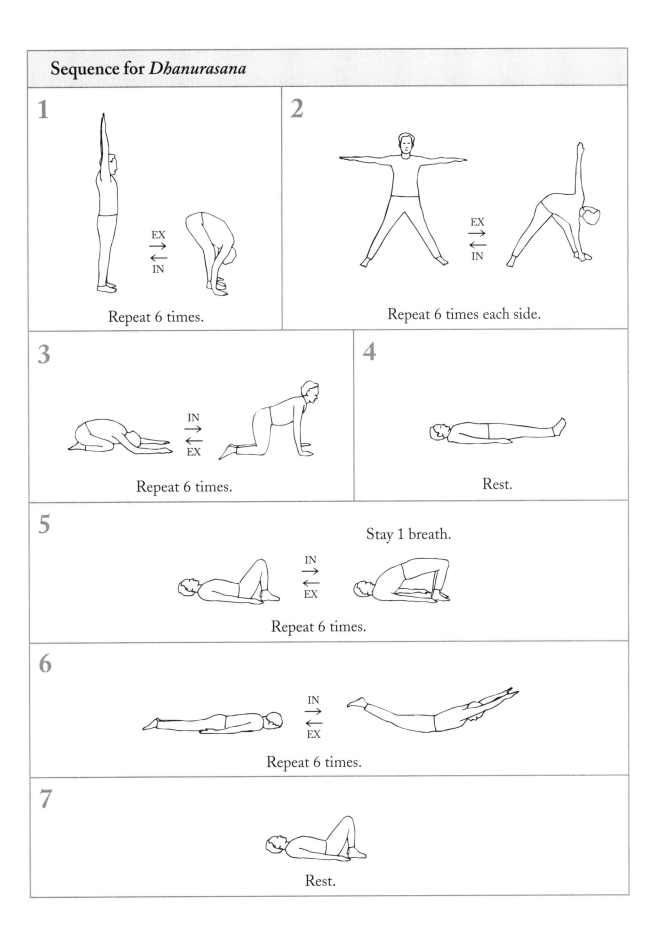

1 Repeat 6 times.

2 Repeat 6 times each side.

3 Repeat 6 times.

4 Rest.

5 Stay 1 breath. Repeat 6 times.

6 Repeat 6 times.

7 Rest.

Sequence for *Dhanurasana* (continued)

8

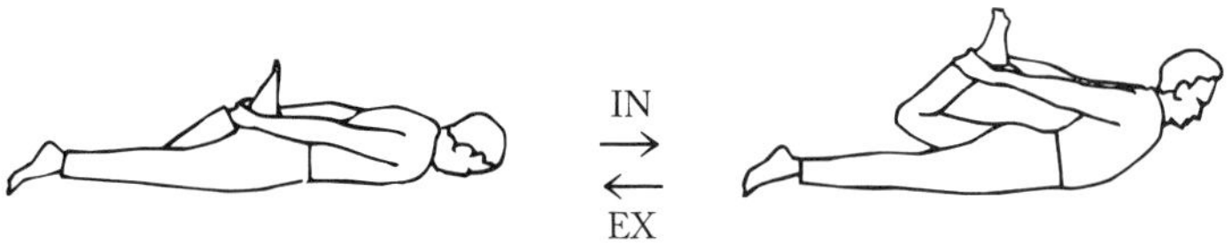

IN →
← EX

Repeat 6 times each side.

9

Stay 3 breaths once.

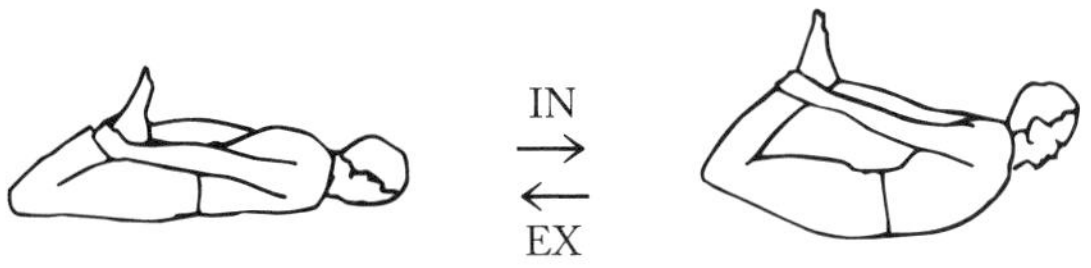

IN →
← EX

Repeat 6 times.

10

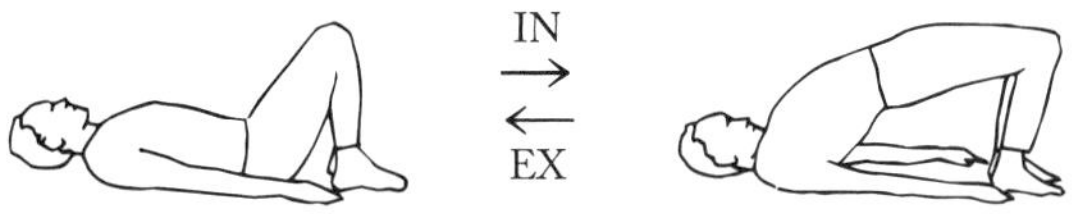

IN →
← EX

Repeat 6 times.

11

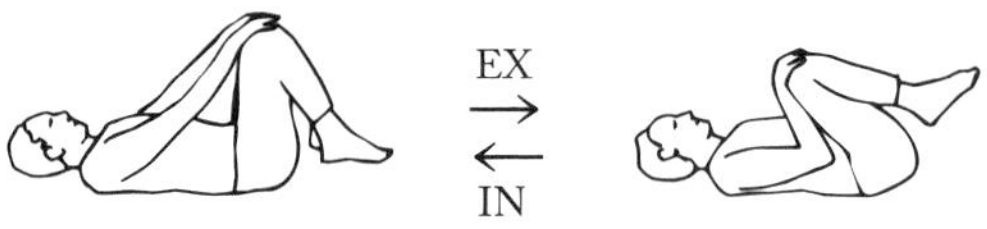

EX →
← IN

Repeat 6 times.

12

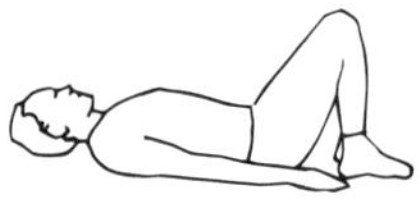

Rest.

Preparation for dvipada viparitakarani. Let us take another difficult asana: *dvipada viparitakarani*. Below we trace the steps a person goes through to do this asana correctly. This sequence of steps is illustrated in figure 4.7.

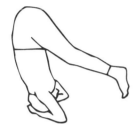

dvipada viparitakarani

1. Essential preparations as listed below
   a. Preparations for shoulder stand such as:
      i. *Uttanasana*: observation of the breath while staying in this position where the head is again lower than the trunk to determine whether the person is ready to progress to more strenuous inverted asanas
      ii. *Adhomukhasvanasana*: head is placed below the trunk in this asana, thus preparing for inversions
      iii. *Dvipadapitham*: to prepare the neck for shoulder stand
   b. Preparation for lowering and raising the legs: *urdhvaprasrtapadasana*
   c. Asanas to develop strength and flexibility of the back: *ardha uttanasana* and *pascimatanasana*
2. Shoulder stand and its variations (a simpler inverted asana)
   a. Simple shoulder stand

   b. Lowering one leg and then both legs in shoulder stand, keeping them bent
   c. Lowering one leg and then both legs in shoulder stand, keeping them straight
3. Headstand (of which the final asana is a variation)
   a. Simple headstand
   b. Lowering each leg separately in headstand, keeping it bent
   c. Lowering both legs in headstand, keeping them bent
   d. Lowering one leg in headstand, keeping it straight
4. The final asana, *dvipada viparitakarani*: lowering both legs to the front from headstand, keeping them straight (the toes do not touch the floor)

Preparation for uttana mayurasana *and* urdhva dhanurasana. The asanas *uttana mayurasana* and *urdhva dhanurasana* have some similarities, but they differ in some areas. Figure 4.8

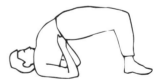

uttana mayurasana

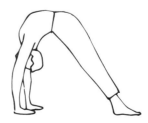

urdhva dhanurasana

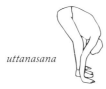

uttanasana

Testing breathing with the head lowered (as preparation for subsequent inversions).

adhomukhasvanasana

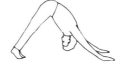

A more intense preparation for inverted positions.

dvipadapitham

Preparing the neck for shoulder stand.

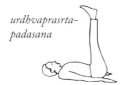

urdhvaprasrta-padasana

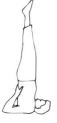

Preparing the abdominal muscles for raising and lowering the legs.

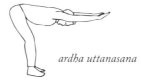

ardha uttanasana

Developing strength in the back.

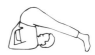

pascimatanasana

Stretching the back to increase flexibility.

STAGE I: PREPARATORY ASANAS

Staying in shoulder stand and breathing comfortably.

Lowering one leg, then both legs, keeping the legs bent.

Lowering one leg, then both legs, keeping the legs straight.

STAGE II: SHOULDER STAND AND ITS VARIATIONS

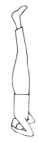

Staying in headstand and breathing comfortably.

Lowering one leg, then both legs, keeping the legs bent.

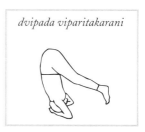

dvipada viparitakarani

Lowering one leg, then both legs, keeping the legs straight.

STAGE III: HEADSTAND AND ITS VARIATIONS

Fig. 4.7. The steps in preparing for *dvipada viparitakarani*.

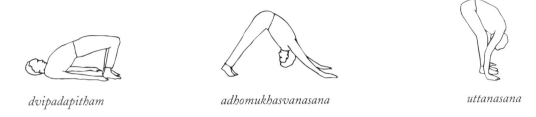

dvipadapitham   *adhomukhasvanasana*   *uttanasana*

Fig. 4.8. Three preparatory asanas for both *uttana mayurasana* and *urdhva dhanurasana*

shows asanas that can help prepare for both. An example sequence is given.

Developing Abdominal Muscle Strength

So far we have discussed how to design a sequence to prepare for a particular asana. We will now discuss how to design a sequence for a particular purpose. There is really no difference between the two. In both cases, the guiding principle is the same—a consideration of the effect of the movements and breathing in the asanas. The preparatory movements for an asana are decided based on the work involved in the asana. The form of the asanas is relevant only in that it is a guide to their effect.

The purpose of this sequence is to build abdominal muscle strength. Figure 5.1 (see page 107) presents a series of movements that demand increasing levels of abdominal muscle strength. Each person can be placed at one of those levels.

The sequence given here is for a healthy young adult. It does not begin at the simplest stage. That would be ineffectual—rather like asking a weight lifter to start training every day using two-pound weights. To start from where the person is, we not only respect the person's weaknesses but also take advantage of his or her strengths. Therefore, we use a few other movements, in the form of some other simpler asanas, to warm up and to prepare all relevant parts of the body and then include the appropriate movements for that person. Over time, we gradually increase the intensity of the movements.

Stretching the Hamstrings and Back

This sequence is of forty-five minutes' duration and is designed for a fit thirty-year-old person with stiffness in the hamstrings and back.

Sequence for *Uttana Mayurasana* and *Urdhva Dhanurasana*

1

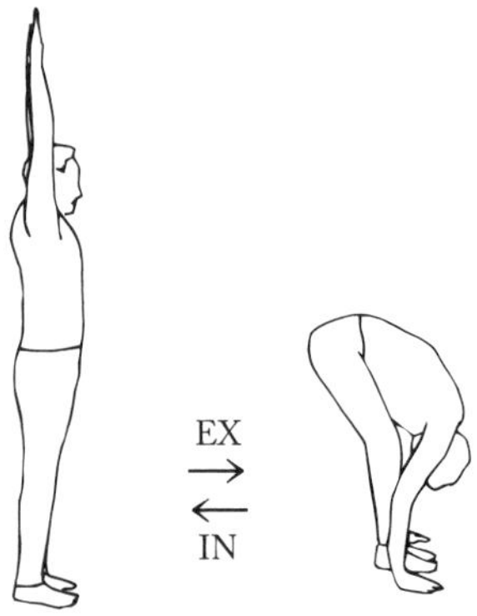

EX →
← IN

Repeat 3 times. Stay 2 breaths once.

2

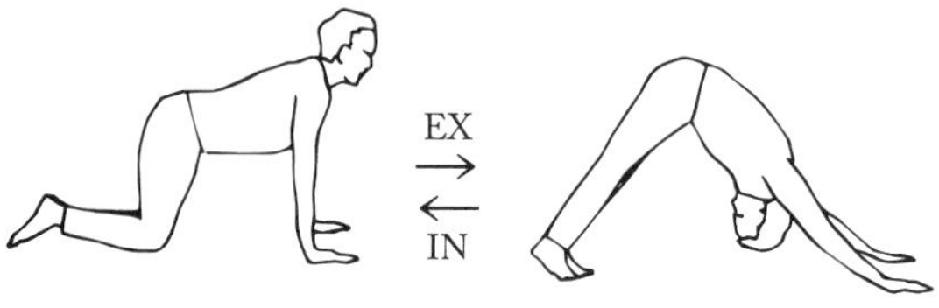

EX →
← IN

Repeat 6 times. Stay 1 breath each time.

3

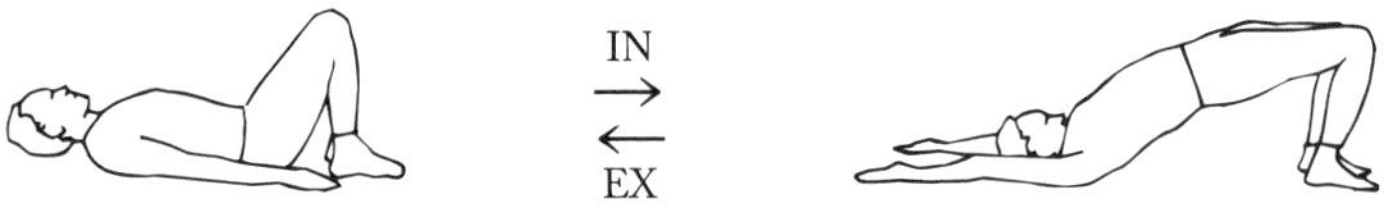

IN →
← EX

Repeat 6 times. Stay 1 breath each time.

4

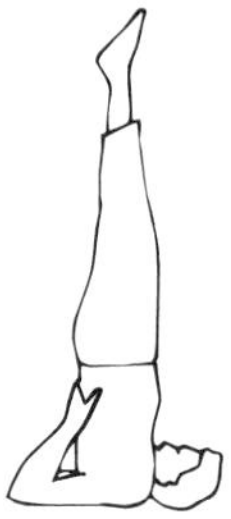

Stay 6 breaths.

5

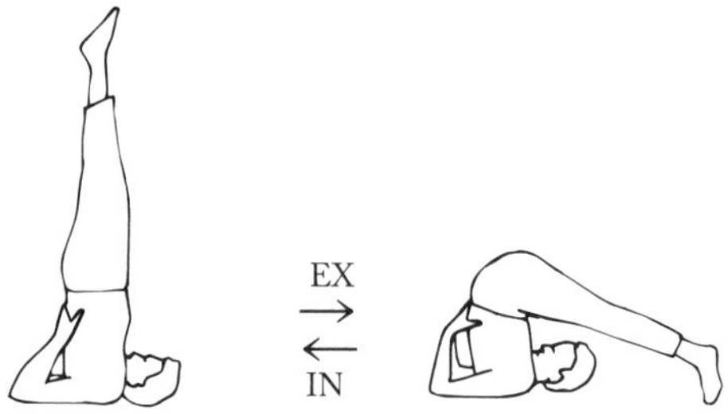

EX →
← IN

Repeat 2 times. Stay 2 breaths each time.

6

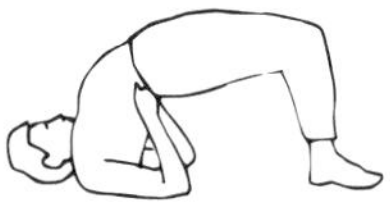

Stay 6 breaths. Free breathing.

7

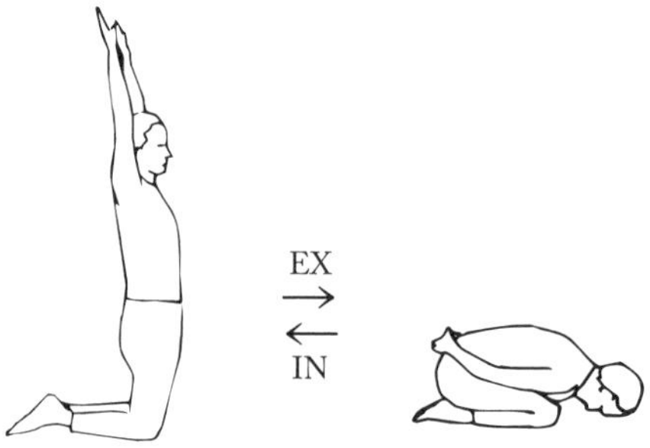

EX →
← IN

Repeat 6 times.

Sequence for *Uttana Mayurasana* and *Urdhva Dhanurasana* (continued)

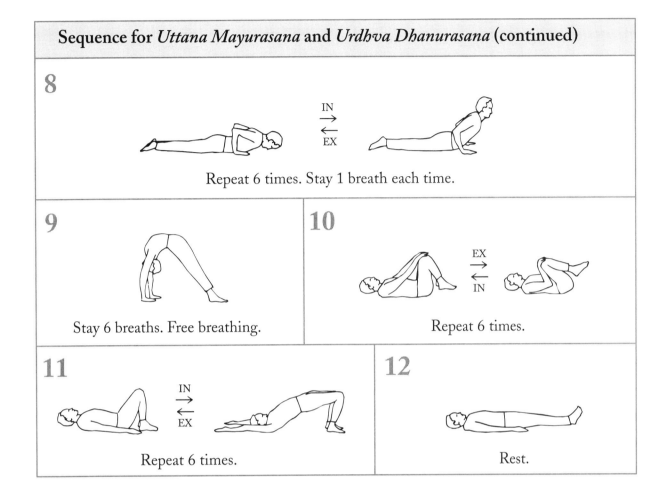

8

IN →
EX ←

Repeat 6 times. Stay 1 breath each time.

9

Stay 6 breaths. Free breathing.

10

EX →
IN ←

Repeat 6 times.

11

IN →
EX ←

Repeat 6 times.

12

Rest.

Developing Abdominal Muscle Strength

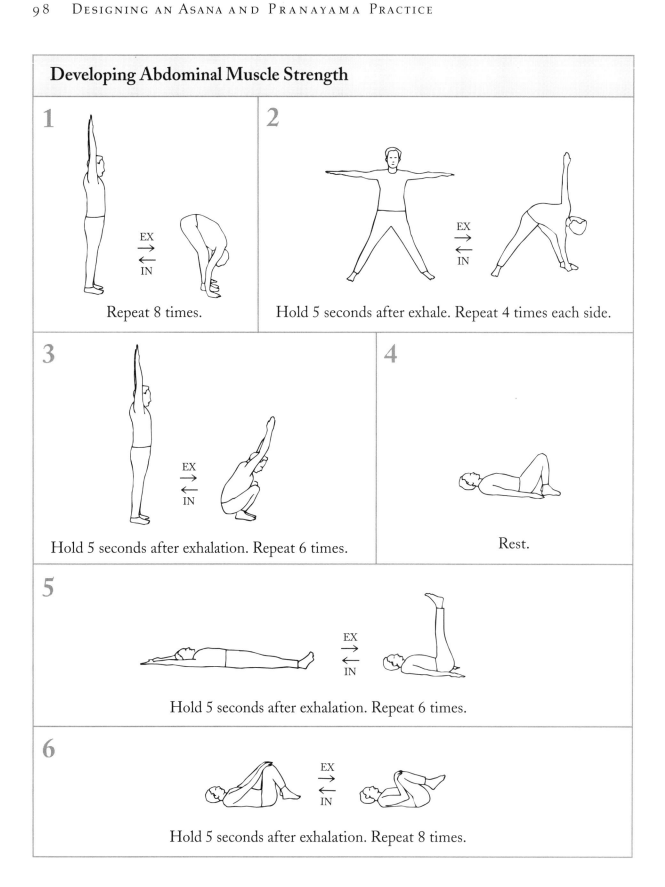

1 Repeat 8 times.

2 Hold 5 seconds after exhale. Repeat 4 times each side.

3 Hold 5 seconds after exhalation. Repeat 6 times.

4 Rest.

5 Hold 5 seconds after exhalation. Repeat 6 times.

6 Hold 5 seconds after exhalation. Repeat 8 times.

Developing Abdominal Muscle Strength (continued)

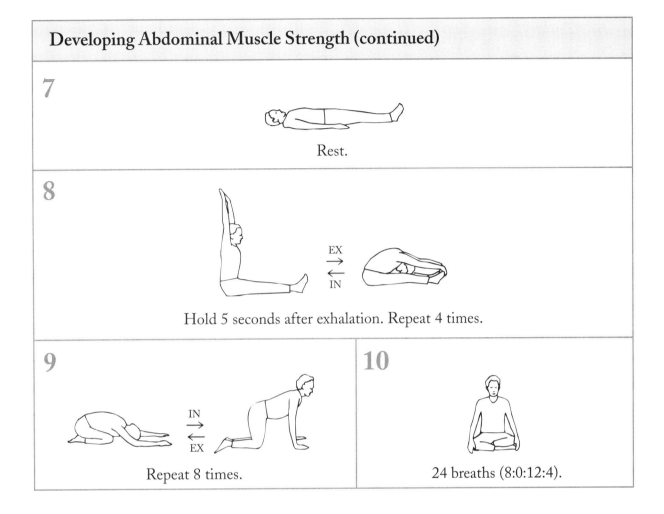

7

Rest.

8

$$\text{EX} \rightarrow$$
$$\leftarrow \text{IN}$$

Hold 5 seconds after exhalation. Repeat 4 times.

9

$$\text{IN} \rightarrow$$
$$\leftarrow \text{EX}$$

Repeat 8 times.

10

24 breaths (8:0:12:4).

Stretching the Hamstrings and Back

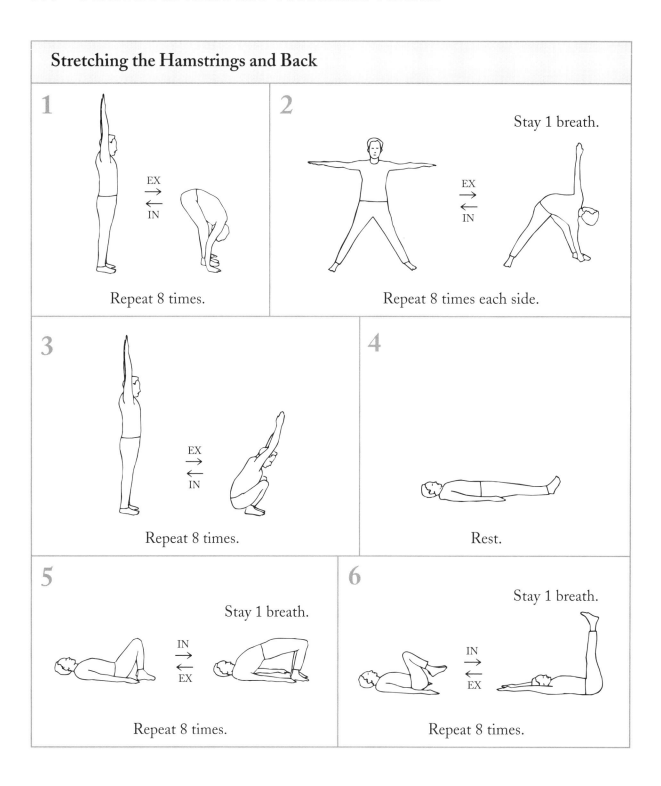

1

EX →
← IN

Repeat 8 times.

2

Stay 1 breath.

EX →
← IN

Repeat 8 times each side.

3

EX →
← IN

Repeat 8 times.

4

Rest.

5

Stay 1 breath.

IN →
← EX

Repeat 8 times.

6

Stay 1 breath.

IN →
← EX

Repeat 8 times.

Stretching the Hamstrings and Back (continued)

7

IN
→
←
EX

Stay 1 breath.

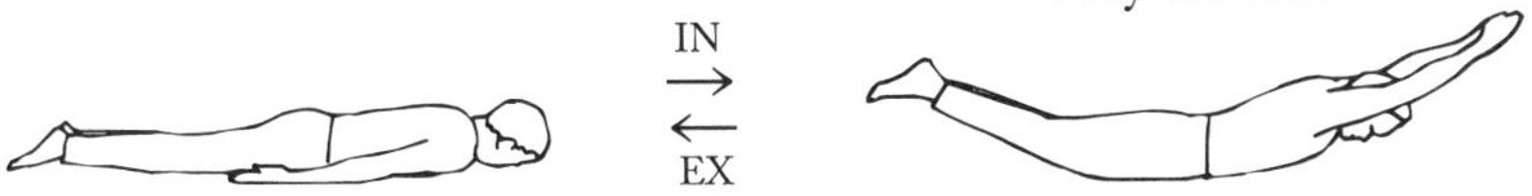

Repeat 8 times.

8

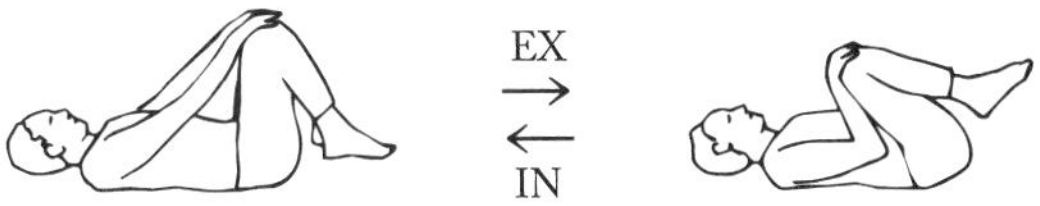

EX
→
←
IN

Repeat 8 times.

9

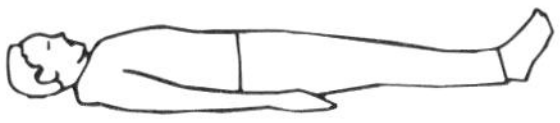

Rest.

Preparation for Kapalabhati Pranayama

Kapalabhati pranayama is rapid breathing done through the nostrils. It involves rapid, strong contraction of the lower abdomen. There are several conditions for which this type of breathing is contraindicated, and therefore it must be practiced and taught carefully. We do not deal with the methodology of teaching or doing the pranayama. We examine the essential aspects that must be considered when we design an asana practice to prepare a person for this pranayama.

You must have good health and stamina before you practice kapalabhati. You must also prepare your abdomen, neck, and nostrils for this pranayama.

The abdomen: This pranayama involves rapid in-and-out movement of the abdomen. Therefore, the abdominal muscles must be in good shape. Preparing the lower back is also necessary.

The neck: When we do rapid abdominal breathing, we tend to lift our head as if we are gasping for air. This must be avoided, as it can lead to several health problems. Even if the breathing is rapid, control is an essential component of all types of pranayama. Therefore, your head must be kept down when you do kapalabhati pranayama. To prepare for this, you must be able to do *jalandhara bandha* (chin lock). Before doing this, make sure you are comfortable breathing in asanas in which the chin is close to the chest, such as *dvipadapitham*.

The nostrils: The nostrils must be clear and free from any obstruction. It is a bad idea to attempt to breathe forcefully through congested nostrils. The buildup of pressure can result in dizziness. To ensure that you can breathe freely, first make sure that you can breathe in inverted asanas. Shoulder stand is an ideal position for this because it is an inverted asana in which the head is in a chin-lock position.

Preparing for Kapalabhati Pranayama

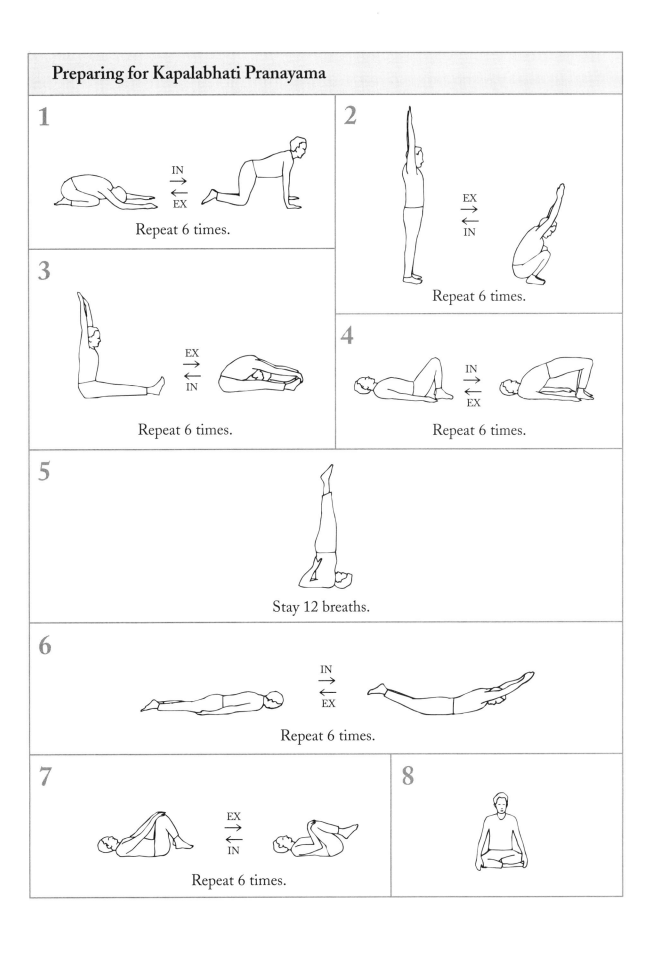

1

IN → ← EX

Repeat 6 times.

2

EX → ← IN

Repeat 6 times.

3

EX → ← IN

Repeat 6 times.

4

IN → ← EX

Repeat 6 times.

5

Stay 12 breaths.

6

IN → ← EX

Repeat 6 times.

7

EX → ← IN

Repeat 6 times.

8

Personalizing the Practice of Asanas

5

PERSONALIZATION MAKES it possible to practice asanas uniquely suited to us. Through observation, we ascertain our needs and assess where we are at present. With our knowledge of the fundamental principles of asana practice, we can decide the general pattern that the movements and breathing should follow. Next, using the principles of sequencing, we design the basic asana practice. Finally, we modify this general plan of movements and breathing, not just so that we can do them but also to maximize their effectiveness.

Health and fitness should be the goal of your asana practice. The ideal form of the asanas is of little importance. We should never force ourselves into the ideal position depicted for an asana. Using external aids to force the body into the position that the "ideal asana" demands is pointless and could even lead to injury. It is not correct to say that all external aids are useless, but the reason for using them must be clear: We must look to the asana's effect or purpose, not its form. If we do not have the level of fitness required to remain in the position reasonably comfortably and do long and smooth breathing, we should not be in that asana at all. Instead, the asana must be modified to make it easier for us to do it.

ACCOMMODATING PROGRESS

Personalization must continuously make room for progress. The practice should not be so simple as to be static. Respecting limits is important, but so is gradually widening them.

Personalizing your practice does not just mean making your practice simple. It can also mean making your practice more strenuous. The pace at which you progress is determined by your condition and diligence, but progress must always be present.

In the practice of asanas, we start from one body position and move into a different one. We generally name the end position as some specific asana. We only need to select a starting position and determine the characteristics of the movement. The end position will automatically fall into place. That is, the final asana is a consequence of working toward the objective, which should be defined in terms of physical or mental health. The effort involved in the movement and breathing combined with our mental state are the most important factors that affect our progress.

Sequencing is a core component in any asana practice because the principles in sequencing are essential to ensure that we continue to make progress. Asanas need to be woven into a cohesive whole that not only serves the immediate purpose but allows us to look forward to the long-term goals as well. Sequencing allows us to do this. After designing a sequence, we need to make refinements to each step so that the practice is optimized for the person. This is the role of personalization. Personalization means that we base our choice of movements and breathing not only on our objectives but on our present needs as well. Personalization makes it possible for each of us to move toward our goal.

Let us look a little deeper into the need for personalization. We all possess structural, physiological, and psychological wellness, but to varying degrees. If you observe any marker of fitness in a number of people, you will find that it is present along a continuum from the extremely feeble to the exceptionally fit.

For example, consider figure 5.1, which illustrates some movements and breathing, ranging from simple to strenuous, that contract the abdominal muscles. In between each of these steps, there can be many more. All such steps or stages are our creations. In reality, what exists is only a continuum along which the strength of contraction gradually increases. We select certain points on this continuum as steps for our use. Asanas themselves are such selections. The body can be in any position that is humanly possible. We choose some of these to be useful as reference points to work from and call them asanas.

To look again at figure 5.1, we all have abdominal muscles that are capable of contracting, and so all of us, except for the very ill, are capable of performing at least some of these movements. Therefore, we all fit somewhere in this range. Our position is decided by the strength of the movements we can and should do, which in turn depends on the strength of our abdominal muscles and other body structures involved in making this movement. A bodybuilder may find a place at the upper end, while an elderly convalescent or a woman a week after childbirth may be at the lower end.

This principle is applicable to any physical

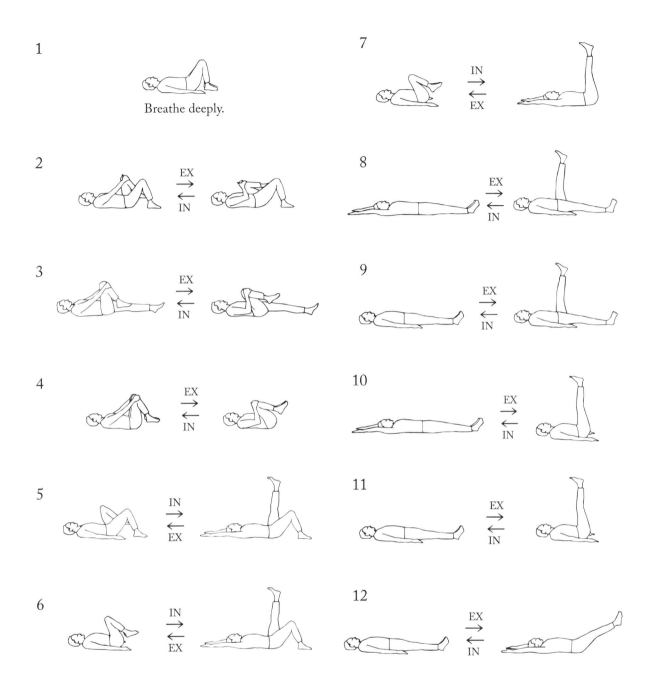

Fig. 5.1. A series of movements requiring increasing abdominal muscle contraction.

or mental function. There always exists a continuum of possibilities starting from the very gentle and extending to the exceptionally strong. In personalization we start with the level that is most suitable for us in our current state of fitness and progress to the more intense levels.

TECHNIQUES OF PERSONALIZATION

Asana practice involves movement of particular parts of the body from a suitable base in a specific direction with an appropriate amount of force over a measured length of time. We can change any or all of these characteristics to produce various effects. We can list these characteristics of movements in asanas as follows:

- *Mula* (base)
- *Desha* (part)
- *Kala* (time)
- *Shakti* (force)
- *Marga* (direction)

It is useful to remember that asanas are composite movements, consisting of a combination of several individual movements. Changes can be made to any of the individual movements. In practice, this means that countless variations are possible. This is why ancient yoga texts say that there are as many asanas as there are living beings.

Mula: The Base

The base and the center of gravity play an important role in any asana. Figure 5.2 shows several examples of how increasing and decreasing the base in asanas alters their effect. Decreasing the base makes it more difficult to maintain balance and consequently makes the asana more challenging. We often use this technique when teaching asanas to children, to keep them interested.

Conversely, increasing the base increases the stability of the asana. As we have seen, some standard asanas are derivations of others, with the main difference being an alteration in the base. For example, *parsva uttanasana* is an altered form of *uttanasana*, with an important difference being the extension of the base in the forward and backward directions. This allows us to intensify the forward movement in the asana without losing balance. Similarly, the twisting movement in *trikonasana* will be more intense than in *samasthiti* because the base is wider and also because *trikonasana* has an added component of forward bending.

Increasing the base is necessary when you find it difficult to maintain your balance. Seated asanas have the advantage of being very stable. This relieves you of the burden of trying to maintain your balance and allows you to focus on the principal movements in the asana. For instance, if you are elderly or unwell, you could sit on a chair and bend forward rather than bending forward from the standing position.

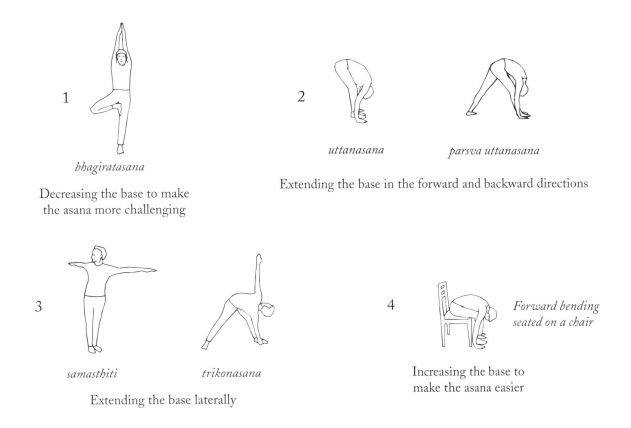

bhagiratasana

Decreasing the base to make
the asana more challenging

uttanasana   *parsva uttanasana*

Extending the base in the forward and backward directions

samasthiti   *trikonasana*

Extending the base laterally

*Forward bending
seated on a chair*

Increasing the base to
make the asana easier

Fig. 5.2. Changes in the base can be made in various asanas to alter their difficulty.

Desha: The Range and Focus of the Movement

The word *desha* literally means "place." In asanas, this involves consideration of the part of the body being moved and the range of the movement.

The range of movement of the head, trunk, arms, or legs can be increased or decreased, with or without the help of external supports. However, restricting the extent of the movement is more common, since many asanas already use the full range of movement possible. In general, the purpose of restricting the range of movement is to make the asana either easier or more difficult. Since we are not altering the movement's basic character, only its extent, the result is more an alteration in the asana's intensity than in the nature of its effect.

Restricting the range of movement to make the asana easier is useful for people who have difficulty doing the complete movement. By progressively increasing the range of

Pushpa, a 40-year-old schoolteacher, is unable to lift her arms overhead. Her neck is stiff, but her back is not weak and her breathing is good.

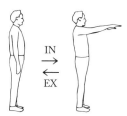

Raise arms up to shoulder level from the front. Stay for 1 breath with the arms raised.

The range of the movement can be increased gradually in subsequent sessions as she progresses. Since her back is not weak and her breathing is good, she can be asked to stay for 1 breath with the arms raised. In an elderly or unfit person, it may be advisable to allow the arms to return to the resting position with each breath.

Paul is a 50-year-old businessman who travels a lot. He often has stiffness in his back.

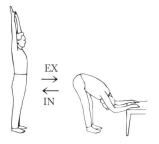

Raise arms on inhalation and bend over on exhalation to rest the hands on a stool. Take a normal breath and return to the standing position on inhalation. Repeat the movement 6 times.

Here we retain the full extent of arm movement but restrict the movement of the trunk because of the stiffness in his back. As before, the range of the movement can be increased over time.

Tara is a 45-year-old housewife. She is overweight and has neck stiffness.

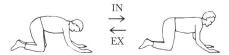

Do not bend down completely. Instead, gently arch the back on each inhalation and round it on exhalation.

Due to her neck stiffness and excess weight, she may find it difficult to bend down completely to rest her head on the floor. Therefore, we restrict the extent of the movement as a whole.

Fig. 5.3. Restricting the range of movement to make an asana easier.

Manfred, 40 years old, practices yoga regularly. His back is strong and he wants to strengthen his abdominal muscles.

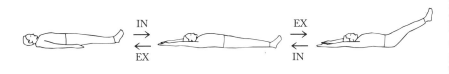

Lie on the back with legs stretched. Raise arms overhead on inhalation. On exhalation, lift the legs a short distance off the floor. Stay for 1 breath and lower the legs on inhalation. Repeat 6 times.

The point of maximum effort in this movement is the initial lifting of the legs off the ground. The effort decreases as the legs move toward a perpendicular position. Therefore, restricting the movement to the initial part intensifies the effort involved. Note that this movement also places the back muscles under a lot of strain, and therefore the person must have strong back muscles before attempting it. Also, he must be very fit, as this is a strenuous exercise.

Ravi is an executive, 38 years old, tall, and well built. He wants to strengthen his back.

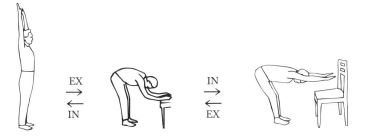

Raise arms on inhalation and bend over on exhalation to rest the arms on a stool. On inhalation, raise arms few inches above the stool. Lower them to the stool on exhalation. Repeat the movement 6 times.

In the movement from the standing position to *uttanasana*, the midway position requires the most effort to hold. Thus, restricting the movement to emphasize that position increases strength.

Fig. 5.4. Restricting the range of movement to make an asana more difficult.

movement as they continue to practice, they may regain the lost function over time (fig. 5.3).

Restricting the extent of the movement can also increase the difficulty of the asana. This can be seen in asanas in which positions between the initial and final position require great effort to stay in. Figure 5.4 shows two common examples.

Apart from modifying the range of the movement, we can also change the movement's focus. That is, we can modify the asana so that it focuses on a different part of the body. Generally, this is achieved by combining

John, a 40-year-old artist, likes to do a few stretches in the morning. He has very tight hamstrings.

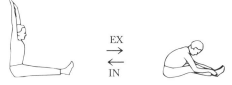

Allow the legs to bend at the knees while bending forward on exhalation and stretch them while returning on inhalation. Repeat the movement 6 to 8 times.

Here we focus the effect on the hamstrings by bending and straightening the legs alternately. The same asana could be used to work on the back. Also, we could achieve the same effect by staying in the final position and using breathing appropriately.

Fig. 5.5. Altering the focus of the movement.

changes in body position with changes in the breathing, as illustrated in figure 5.5.

Kala: The Duration of the Movement

Kala is the time taken for the movement, that is, the duration of the movement. This determines the movement's speed.

We have seen that asanas involve movement into, staying in, and movement out of a position. Each of these is always associated with one of the components of the breathing cycle. Therefore, changing the duration of movement amounts to changing the duration of breathing. We emphasize this because breathing is the factor that should determine the duration of an asana.

Increasing the duration of a movement usually intensifies its effect. We generally discourage doing very fast movements in the practice of asanas, as this increases the risk of injury, disturbs the flow of the breath, and does not calm the mind. Fast movements can be used selectively, in specific situations where such vigorous activity is desirable. Usually it is better to do slow movements with appropriate deep, long, and controlled breathing. This can be effective in increasing strength, stamina, or flexibility, depending on the nature of the asana. Furthermore, this allows sufficient time for the breathing to exert maximum effect. This can be a powerful tool in augmenting the movement's positive effects.

Because of the prominent role of breathing in asanas, this is a very valuable principle. Figure 5.6 illustrates the uses of this principle in *uttanasana*. Figure 5.7 gives some examples of the application of this principle to specific situations.

Shakti: The Force behind the Movement

Shakti is the force behind the movement. The force required to make movements can be increased by adding to the load in the asana. This can be done using external aids: holding books or even weights in the hands

	Movement	Modification	Effect or Purpose
1		Bend down very slowly with extended exhalation.	Gradually increasing, sustained stretching of the hamstrings.
2		Return to the standing position very slowly, with extended inhalation.	Done with emphasis on the spine, this works strongly to straighten the upper back.
3		Stay in the final position with suspension after exhalation.	Strengthening of the abdominal muscles.
4		Repeat 12 times with short inhalation and exhalation.	Warming up.
5		Hold 5 seconds after inhalation.	Improving chest breathing.

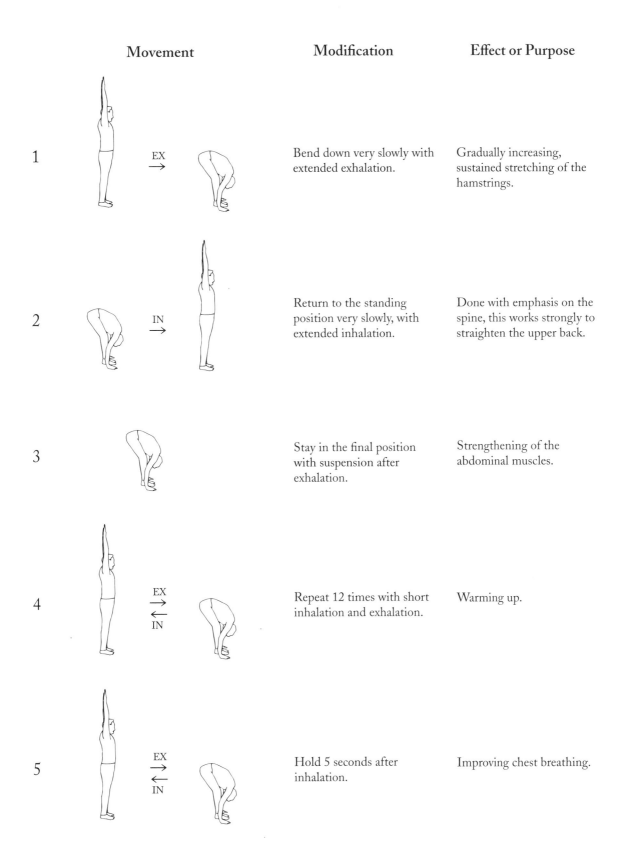

Fig. 5.6. Modifying the duration of the movement by using breathing.

Tom, 36 years old, is used to regular exercise. He wants to increase his stamina.

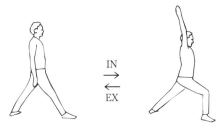

Hold the breath for 5 seconds after inhalation. Exhale freely.

Staying in positions that require strength, with extension of breathing, is an effective way to develop stamina.

Harris, 40 years old, works in an advertising firm. He is highly stressed and wants to relax and feel well in the evening.

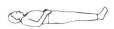

Lie down with legs stretched out and relaxed, hands on the abdomen. Close the eyes and focus on the exhalation, lengthening it as much as possible. Stay for 12 breaths.

The focus is on breathing—the extended exhalation. Combined with the relaxed position of the body, it helps to calm the mind and reduce stress.

Meena, 29 years old, has a 10-month-old baby. She did not exercise after delivery, and her abdominal muscles lack strength.

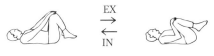

Lie down with legs bent, with the hands holding the knees. Bring the knees toward the chest while exhaling. Pause for 5 seconds after completing exhalation. On inhalation, move the legs away from the chest. Repeat 6 to 8 times.

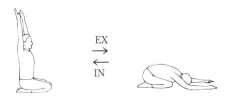

Bend the legs and sit on the heels. Raise the arms on inhalation. Bend over on exhalation to rest the head and arms on the floor. Pause for 5 seconds after exhalation. On inhalation, raise the arms and return to the initial position. Repeat 6 to 8 times.

Suspension after exhalation helps in contracting the abdominal muscles. The flexed position of the body aids in this. This is a gentle means to work on the abdominal muscles, mainly by using the breathing. We can suggest progressively stronger movements as her abdominal muscle strength improves with continued practice.

Fig. 5.7. Altering the duration of the movement.

or between the legs (fig. 5.8). Usually, external aids are used to increase the force in an asana in cases where a fit person wishes to build more strength. Alternatively, the weight of the body can be redistributed to make the movement less or more strenuous. Altering the position of body parts to reduce the load in an asana is particularly useful in therapeutic situations if the person finds the normal asana difficult or demanding.

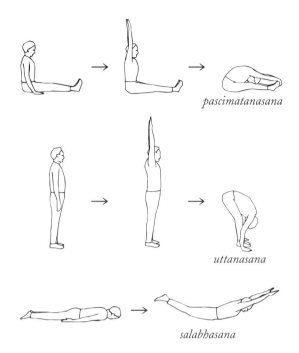

pascimatanasana

uttanasana

salabhasana

Marga: The Direction of the Movement

Marga is the direction in which the movement is made. As we have seen, asanas include movement in all three planes, allowing us maximum flexibility in choosing the direction of the movements we wish to make. Every asana is characterized by specific principal movements and particular body positions. For instance, in *uttanasana*, the principal movement is a forward-bending movement at the hips, done from the standing position. *Pascimatanasana* involves a similar movement done from a seated position.

Salabhasana involves extension of the trunk done from the prone position. In all asanas, apart from the principal movement, which usually concerns the trunk, there are accessory movements of the other parts of the body such as the head, arms, and legs. In *uttanasana* and *pascimatanasana*, for example, the forward-bending movement is preceded by raising the arms, which then remain in an

Robert, 30 years old, is a marathon runner. He wants to strengthen his back muscles.

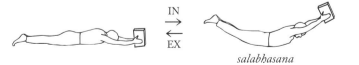

IN
→
←
EX

salabhasana

Hold book in hands when doing *salabhasana*. A book could be held between the legs as well.

Since Robert is very fit, using external aids is appropriate for him. In other cases, it may be safer to extend the movement with an emphasis on inhalation.

Fig. 5.8. Using external aids to alter the force required for the movement.

extended position throughout the movement. In *salabhasana*, the raising of the arms is done at the same time as the principal movement.

Changing the direction of the principal movement—and sometimes the position of the body—will transform one asana into another and consequently may create a completely different effect. In that case, we are not modifying the asana; we are simply using another. But the accessory movements can be changed to modify the effect of the asana; this falls under personalization (fig. 5.9).

Using Supports and External Aids

The purpose of using a support or an external aid is not to force yourself into the classical position depicted for an asana. You must be very clear about why you are using a support—it must help you to gain some attribute of health or to progress further. In other words, the use of a support should help to promote any one or all of the five aspects required for good health mentioned in chapter 2.

Consider the following example. You may have developed the necessary strength, flexi-bility, and coordination to do a headstand and not have any significant spinal misalignment. However, if you are not sure of maintaining your balance, you can start by using the wall for support. In time, you will gain the confidence required to do a headstand without the support of the wall. But if you suspend your-self in an inverted position using platforms or other mechanisms, you need to ask yourself if you are truly gaining greater health by this. Will this help you develop greater strength, flexibility, or coordination? Will this ever lead you to do a headstand properly? Also, if your body is not prepared to be in an inverted body position, you will definitely find it uncomfort-able to breathe when you are upside down. Will forcing yourself into an unfamiliar body position without adequate preparation improve your health? Would it not be better to start with simpler forms of inversion, even as simple as lying down with your feet raised onto a support like a chair, and doing deep extended breathing that can calm your mind, improve your breathing capacity, and benefit the functioning of various body systems? Try both methods and experience the difference for yourself.

Peter, 43 years old, has neck stiffness after doing headstand.

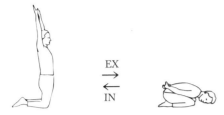

Kneel down and raise the arms on inhalation. Bend forward and downward, sweeping the arms backward and turning the head to one side. Repeat the movement 3 times on each side.

The principal movement in this asana (*vajrasana*) is the forward-bending movement at the hips, done from the kneeling position. The arms and head are free to move and we can alter the direction of their movement. Usually we allow the head to remain in line with the trunk, facing downward in the final position. In this case, we turn the head from side to side in alternate repetitions to relax and stretch the neck muscles and relieve stiffness. Sweeping the arms to the back (instead of resting them in front, by the side of the head) also aids in this.

Mani, 38 years old, has asymmetry in his shoulders. His back is strong and he is used to exercise.

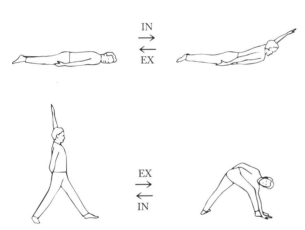

Lie on the stomach with the hands by the side and the head turned to one side. On inhalation, raise the trunk, sweeping one arm forward and straightening the head. On exhalation, lower the trunk, sweeping the arms backward and turning the head to the opposite side. Repeat 3 times on each side.

In the initial position, raise one arm on inhalation. Bend forward on exhalation, turning the head to one side in the end position. Repeat the movement 6 times on each side.

Here we move the arms alternately and turn the head to work on each side of the neck and shoulders separately.

Fig. 5.9. Altering the direction of the movement.

Pranayama 6

FROM ASANAS TO PRANAYAMA

In asanas, the emphasis is on the movement of the body. The breath is an aid. That is, movements of the body cannot be done without affecting the flow of the breath; and the flow of the breath in turn affects the structure and function of the body. Therefore, whenever we move our body in asana practice, we take into consideration this link and use the breath to support or aid the movement rather than oppose it.

In pranayama, we focus exclusively on changing the pattern of breathing, tailoring it to a particular individual for a specific purpose. Here we change the movement of the breath, while remaining in a particular posture. The most important role of the body in the practice of pranayama lies in not disturbing the flow of the breath or the focus of the mind.

The body and breath are inseparably interwoven. Therefore, it is incorrect to classify the practice of asanas and pranayama as working solely with the body and breath, respectively. The difference lies in the degree of emphasis. In asana, the principal focus is on the achievement of strength and flexibility, though not without attention to the state of mind. The primary means is the movement of the body, with the breath playing a supporting role in enhancing the benefit of the movement. In the practice of pranayama, the principal focus is on the achievement of mental steadiness. The primary means is the active regulation of breathing, with the body playing a supporting role in providing a firm and comfortable position for the practice.

TABLE 6.1. Comparison of asana and pranayama.

Asana	Pranayama
There are four parts of body movement: • Arm • Trunk • Leg • Head	There are four components of the movement of breath: • Inhalation • Retention • Exhalation • Suspension
There are four directions of movement.	There are different methodologies of breathing.
There are four basic body positions.	The postures are seated or lying, with proper mental focus.
There are different possible combinations of movement and breath. These give rise to various asanas. There are orderly steps (*vinyasa-krama*) for each asana.	There are different possible combinations of components and types of breathing. These constitute the various types and ratios in pranayama. There are orderly steps (*vinyasa-krama*) for each pranayama.
Each movement has a distinct nature. These movements are related, and one affects the other. For example, arm movement affects the trunk.	Each component of breath has a distinct nature. Different components of breath affect each other. For example, long exhalation can affect inhalation.
We use breath to make our body strong and flexible.	We choose the body position to aid the breathing pattern.
Asanas can be arranged for a purpose—to do a posture or fulfill a particular need.	Pranayama can be varied for a purpose—to do a particular ratio or recover from sickness.
We need to observe and personalize the practice for the person.	We need to observe and personalize the practice for the person.

Pranayama also has therapeutic applications through influencing specific doshas.

Pranayama is the fourth limb in Patanjali's eight limbs of yoga. It can be regarded as the link between the external and the internal practices of yoga. This is significant because breath is the link between the body and the mind. Table 6.1 provides a comparison of asana and pranayama.

THE MEANING OF PRANAYAMA

What Is Prana?

The word *prana* occurs frequently in Vedic literature. The meaning of this word, however, varies in different contexts. We will discuss below three important meanings of this word.

Prana in the Vedas. Prana is an intrinsic property of the Seer, or consciousness. It is the power of the Seer to cause the functions of life to proceed in its presence. It is responsible for the functioning of the mind and the body, including the senses. Prana is present because of the Seer, and therefore it exists in all living things.

Prana is not air. We cannot acquire more prana from outside by breathing it into our bodies. Prana is beyond sense perception because it is the reason the senses function at all. Prana cannot be directly cognized or experienced even at the level of the mind for the simple reason that it is what is responsible for the mind's ability to cognize or experience. The very existence of prana is an inference, not a direct experience. What we experience is the functioning of the mind, body, and senses as a consequence of the existence of prana. Prana exists even in deep sleep when we have no conscious experience; it is the reason the body continues to function while we sleep.

It is important to understand that prana does not have an existence independent of the Seer. It is not a force that has direct physical expression like gravity or electrostatic force. The expression of the existence of prana is only through the function of the body and mind.

When we talk about the flow of prana being impaired in any part of the body, what is implied is an impairment of normal life functions in that part of the body. Conversely, the proper flow of prana means that all aspects of the body and the mind function properly; that is, there is health. As we have discussed, the nature of prana means that it is impossible to manipulate it directly to restore its function, without reference to the body or mind. The tools we have at our disposal are the body, the breath, the mind, and food. Using these, we can restore or improve the functioning of the body and mind. This restoration of optimum function is, as we have stated, the restoration of the proper flow of prana. Roughly speaking, we use asanas, pranayama, meditation, and Ayurveda to work with body, breath, mind, and food, respectively, to restore or maintain the proper flow of prana. In this way we can regain or maintain health.

We infer the existence of prana only because of the existence of movement—of the body, breath, or mind. A disturbance of these movements reflects a disturbance of the movement or flow of prana. Consequently, we change the movements of the body, breath, and mind appropriately to rectify or restore the movement of the prana.

Prana in Ayurveda. Ayurveda is based on the theory of the three doshas: Vata, Pitta, and Kapha. Each has five divisions. Prana vata is one of the divisions of Vata. Prana vata is responsible for a subset of the functions of Vata. Prana in the previous definition is essential for all life functions, for the functioning of all the doshas, while prana vata as defined in Ayurveda is only one of the components of the Vata dosha. Prana vata is not the breath. Breathing is the result of the function of prana vata in the upper region of the body. One of the most important functions of prana vata is to cause the movement responsible for breathing.

Prana in yoga. Philosophically, the concept of prana in yoga is the same as that in the Upanishads: It is the power of the Seer. When referring to practical techniques such as pranayama, however, some texts such as the *Hatha-Yoga-Pradipika* use the term *prana vayu.* The word *vayu* refers to the external air. Prana vayu is nothing but the air we breathe in and out. Sometimes, the word *vayu* is dropped and just the word *prana* is used. The air we breathe is the most important and obvious necessity for the sustenance of life, and thus words such as *prana* (life force) or *amrita* (nectar) are sometimes used poetically to refer to it. Therefore, in the word *pranayama, prana* should be taken to refer simply to the breath.

What Is Ayama?

The word *ayama* means "to lengthen or extend." *Pranayama* literally means "to lengthen or extend the prana." Prana as the power of the Seer is, by definition, not subject to such manipulation, and so pranayama means literally "to lengthen the breath."

We measure time based on the movement of the earth on its axis and around the sun. The rotation of the earth on its axis takes one day. This we build up to years and break down to seconds. Based on this time frame, a human being can live for approximately one hundred years. Alternatively, we can measure time in terms of the number of breaths we take in and let out.

Our physical activities and mental state affect our breathing rate. Eating heavy food also increases our breathing rate.

Proper food, meditation, and asana practice make it possible to live a healthy life up to one hundred years of age. In order to reduce our total number of breaths, we do deep breathing in asana practice and in pranayama. It is therefore imperative that we not shorten our breath through jumping from one asana to another or using force in the practice of asanas. This would be counterproductive. As we grow older, this is more important, since the effort needed will be greater and the breathing rate will increase with effort. For older people, pranayama is given more importance, since it directly involves lengthening the breath.

At the physical level, a natural rhythm of fewer breaths per minute in a fit person usually indicates an increased level of respiratory and cardiovascular fitness.

WHY PRANAYAMA?

We listed several goals for the practice of asanas: structural, physiological, and psychological. Asanas encompass a limitless variety of dynamic movements that naturally provide powerful means for maintaining and enhancing structural well-being. In contrast to asanas, the practice of pranayama involves minimizing the movement of the body and focusing on the movement of the breath. Moving the body is discouraged in pranayama, as it can disturb our control over the flow of our breath. Therefore, the focus in pranayama is on achieving physiological and psychological well-being. Breath is a key link between the body and mind, and therefore pranayama is ideally suited to achieving these goals.

The physical goals of pranayama can be either to recover from sickness or to maintain health. At the level of the mind, pranayama aids in achieving a base level of mental balance that will allow us to effectively practice meditation. Asana, pranayama, and meditation—emphasizing the body, breath, and

mind, respectively—are very important practices on the path of yoga.

As with asanas, we need to understand the factors that constitute the practice of pranayama and their characteristics and interconnections, in order to use pranayama to achieve a particular purpose and personalize our practice.

The purpose, means, and result for asanas and pranayama based on the *Yoga-Sutras* are given in table 6.2.

Pranayama is the means to remove mental disturbances and make the mind focused for meditation (*Yoga-Sutras* 2.52, 53). The removal of mental disturbance is achieved by making our breath long, steady, smooth, and subtle (2.50). This in turn is achieved through consciously changing the pattern of our breathing (2.49). There are several aspects involved in making the breath long, steady, smooth, and subtle. These include the posture, the different components of the breathing process, and the mental focus. We will discuss each of these.

THE HOW OF PRANAYAMA

We spend our lives alternating between three states of consciousness: waking, dreaming, and deep sleep. We cannot, of course, be aware of our breathing when we are dreaming or in deep sleep, but even when we are awake, our breathing usually remains an unconscious activity. We become aware of our breathing pattern only when it is disturbed, for example, when we are involved in a physically

TABLE 6.2. Comparison of the purpose, means, and result of asanas and pranayama (based on the *Yoga-Sutras*).

	Asanas	Pranayama
Purpose	To make the body strong and flexible so the posture for pranayama is steady and comfortable (2.46)	To steady the mind by changing the pattern of breathing (2.49)
Means	• Proper movement • Use of breath • Clarity of purpose (2.47)	• Right posture • Active regulation of breath • Proper mental focus (2.50)
Result	Less disturbance from pairs of opposites (2.48)	Reduction of mental colorings (2.52). The mind becomes fit for focus or concentration. (2.53)

demanding activity or when we are emotionally upset.

Disturbances of the body and mind alter the pattern of our breathing (*Yoga-Sutras* 1.31). It is obvious that discomfort in the body disturbs our pattern of breathing. Pain or fever, for instance, affects our normal unconscious breathing pattern. Similarly, the breathing pattern and the flow of thoughts in the mind are intricately linked. Observe someone who is agitated, and you will see that his or her breathing is rapid, short, and often shallow. Observe your own breathing when you are calm and you will see that your breath is longer and smoother than normal.

The length and smoothness of breathing reflect the degree of absorption of the mind. The converse is also true: Consciously increasing the length and smoothness of our breath calms the mind. In pranayama, we deliberately use this connection that breathing has with the mind and body; we consciously change our breathing pattern to reduce bodily imbalance and mental disturbance.

The practice of pranayama is an exceptionally useful tool for bringing about changes in our mind. Our mind has no form distinct from its ceaseless flux of thoughts. Therefore, at the outset it is often difficult to bring about sustained changes in our thought process by working directly with only our mind. It is easier instead to start by working with the breath, for our breathing pattern is more readily observable and more amenable to control.

A change in our pattern of breathing can be brought about by either passive observation of the breath or active regulation of the components of the breathing cycle.

Passive Observation

In passive observation, we allow our mind to become aware of the nature or quality of our breath—inhalation, exhalation, the pauses between them, the length and smoothness of the breath, and so on. But we do not consciously attempt to change any of these characteristics, to alter the pattern of breathing in any way, or to regulate any part of the breathing cycle. We merely stay focused on the present nature of our breath.

As our mind becomes more fully absorbed in observing the flow of the breath, the character of our breathing tends to change involuntarily. Our breath becomes longer and smoother simply because we are aware of it. This change in our breathing in turn exerts a calming influence on the mind, deepening our focus. Thus a positive cycle is set up, reinforcing our mental absorption.

This is, strictly speaking, meditation with the object of focus being the character of the breathing. The abstract nature of the object (the breath) calls for a high degree of awareness for this meditation to be successful.

Active Regulation

Consciously changing the pattern of breathing involves active regulation of the components of the breathing pattern. Each component of the breathing cycle has specific effects on the state of the mind and the body.

We can intelligently use this connection for several purposes: therapeutic, preventive, and others. This versatility is absent in passive observation. Of course, such active regulation can, and ultimately must, be used to bring about long (*dirgha*) and smooth (*sukshma*) breathing. It should also result in a focused mind.

WHAT CONSTITUTES PRANAYAMA?

As a practice, pranayama is the alteration of the flow of the breath together with the focus of the mind. The flow of the breath is a physical process. It occupies a certain period of time. We can focus our mind on any object, including the breath itself, for this period. Thus pranayama consists of three components: physical, mental, and temporal.

1. Physical factors
   • Position of the body: asana for pranayama
   • Four components of the breathing cycle: inhalation, retention, exhalation, and suspension
   • Methodology of breathing: route of entry and exit of air (through the nose or mouth) and other special types of breathing (for example, through a curled tongue in *shitali* pranayama)
2. Mental factor: the focus of the mind (desha)
3. Temporal factors
   • Duration of each of the components of the breathing cycle (kala)

• Total number of repetitions: the duration of the pranayama session as a whole (*samkhya*)

Any pranayama is a combination of these components. The characteristics of the components define each particular type of pranayama. The *Yoga-Sutras* emphasize using pranayama to make the breath long, steady, smooth, and subtle. But whatever the purpose (fitness or therapy), the factors listed above are involved. A clear understanding of their effect and the connections between them is essential. For therapeutic uses, an understanding of the relationship between these factors and the three doshas is also required.

Some important principles of pranayama practice are given below:

1. Components of breathing. We have discussed four components of the breath: inhalation, holding after inhalation, exhalation, and suspension after exhalation. Inhalation and exhalation involve movement, while the other two components are their static extensions. In inhalation or exhalation, the movement has two characteristics that we can alter: the route of entry and exit of the air and the length of the breath.

2. Nose or mouth breathing. There are only two entry or exit points for the breath: the nose and the mouth. Normally, we inhale and exhale through the nose using both nostrils. We can also breathe through only one nostril by closing the other one. For example, we can inhale through the left nostril and

exhale through the right nostril. But we do not exhale through the mouth in the practice of pranayama, as this is said to lead to a loss of energy (*Hatha-Yoga-Pradipika* 2.54, commentary of Brahmananda).

3. Changing the duration of the breathing components. We can consciously alter the duration of any of the components of breathing. We can increase the duration of one or more breathing components to make the breath slower. Alternatively, we can decrease the duration of the breathing components to make the breath faster. To do either in a controlled manner, we need to regulate the flow of the breath either at the throat or at the nostrils.

4. Pranayamas are innumerable. Variations of nose and mouth breathing used in inhalation and exhalation, combined with changes in the duration of the components of the breathing cycle, can yield limitless varieties of pranayama. Thus it is said that pranayamas are innumerable. Some of the types of pranayama presented in classical yoga texts are listed later in this chapter.

5. The importance of mental focus. The flow of the breath is linked to the movement of the mind. Therefore, to derive maximum benefit from the practice of pranayama, it is very important to focus your mind, perhaps on the flow of your breath or on a mantra or a specific region of the body, depending on your purpose and attitude.

6. Posture is an aid to breathing and mental focus. The position of the body and the shape of the spine affect the flow of the

breath. Since we have to remain in one position for the duration of the pranayama practice, it must be stable and comfortable. Otherwise, discomfort in the body will hinder the smooth flow of breath and draw our mind away from the desired focus.

7. Repetition results in the desired effect. In pranayama we seek to regularize or change our disturbed or unconscious pattern of breathing through conscious effort. Any sustained changes that will produce significant results can be achieved only over a number of repetitions or cycles.

Posture for Pranayama

The *Yoga-Sutras* do not recommend any particular posture for pranayama. They merely stipulate that pranayama should be done "after having mastered a posture," the posture being one that is stable and comfortable. This is a logical approach, since the posture will vary based on the person and purpose. Pranayama can be done standing, lying down, or seated on the floor or on a chair. Some classical yoga texts such as the *Hatha-Yoga-Pradipika* recommend seated postures like *padmasana*, *sukhasana*, *vajrasana*, *brahmasana*, *svastikasana*, or *siddhasana* (fig. 6.1). In pranayama for therapy, we may use much more comfortable postures (fig. 6.2).

Here are some practical guidelines (especially for pranayama in the seated position):

- Keep your spine erect.
- Assess your normal breathing before commencing the practice of pranayama. If the posture is appropriate, the flow of breathing in pranayama should be as easy and smooth as normal breathing.
- Choose the correct posture. Otherwise, your breathing could become strained over a number of cycles.
- Make sure your abdomen and chest are free of tension to allow the free flow of breath.
- Choose a posture in which you can breathe freely with attention.

External supports may be required to make the posture stable and comfortable and

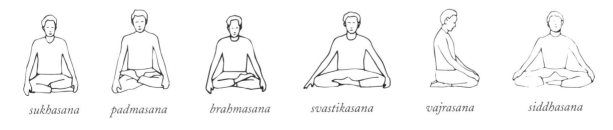

sukhasana   *padmasana*   *brahmasana*   *svastikasana*   *vajrasana*   *siddhasana*

Fig. 6.1. Postures recommended for pranayama in ancient yoga texts.

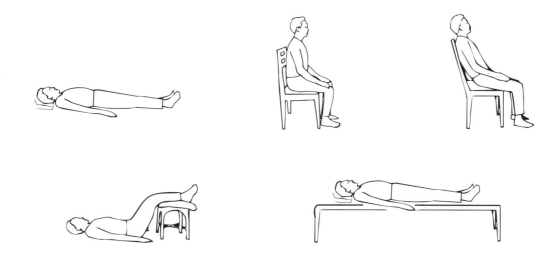

Fig. 6.2. Postures for pranayama, modified for use in therapeutic situations.

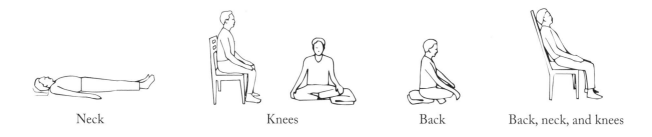

Neck   Knees   Back   Back, neck, and knees

Fig. 6.3. The back, neck, or knees may need support when practicing pranayama.

fulfill these guidelines. The purpose of using supports is to minimize discomfort that may interfere with the smooth flow of breath or disturb the focus of the mind.

The back, neck, and knees are usually the areas of our body needing support (fig. 6.3). Observation during our asana practice can help to determine which areas need support.

Asanas as Preparation for Pranayama

Asanas help to prepare the body and the breath for the practice of pranayama in the following ways:

- Determining the best posture for pranayama based on observation of asana practice

- Preparing the body to remain seated for an extended time in that posture
- Determining the breathing ratio to be used in the practice of pranayama and preparing for that ratio
- Focusing the mind
- Preparing for the bandhas
- Balancing the effect of long sitting after the practice of pranayama

The following steps are involved in preparation:

- Choose the posture.
- Prepare the body to stay comfortably for the required length of time in that posture.
- Simultaneously prepare the breath to flow smoothly in the ratio chosen.
- Assume the posture.
- If necessary, perform appropriate simple movements to open out the chest and relax the abdomen and back. Use breathing with ratios leading to those to be practiced.
- Rest, observe the breath, and then start the practice of pranayama.

Two examples are illustrated in figure 6.4.

The Breathing Cycle

The breathing cycle consists of four components:

- Exhalation: the outward movement of the breath (*recaka*)
- Inhalation: the inward movement of the breath (*puraka*)
- Suspension of the breath after exhalation (*bahya-kumbhaka*)
- Retention of the breath after inhalation (*antar-kumbhaka*)

The characteristics of each of these are discussed in detail in my book *Yoga for Body, Breath, and Mind*.

The quality of one's pranayama practice is to be judged by the smoothness, steadiness, and length of the breath and the focus of the mind. The volume of air moving in and out of the lungs is not the criterion for judging the quality of the practice.

Exhalation. Pranayama is a means to reduce disturbance in the mind. Conscious smooth and long exhalation is the most effective means to achieve this (*Yoga-Sutras* 1.34). Such extended exhalation reduces rajas (hyperactivity), thus calming the mind. At the physical level, extended exhalation works on the lower abdomen. It brings about lightness in the body.

The duration and quality of the exhalation is the most important factor to be considered when we are choosing the ratios of the breathing components for pranayama. Also, since inhalation and exhalation are the two complementary phases of the cyclic breathing process, extended exhalation promotes deeper and fuller inhalation.

Inhalation. Inhalation, like eating, is a process of taking in, while exhalation is one of elimination. As with eating, inhalation should be limited to the amount necessary. Just as it is

Steps	Example 1	Example 2
Decide on the posture.	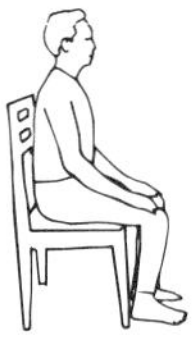	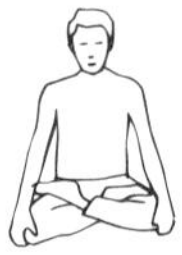
Prepare the body to sit in the posture.	No preparation needed.	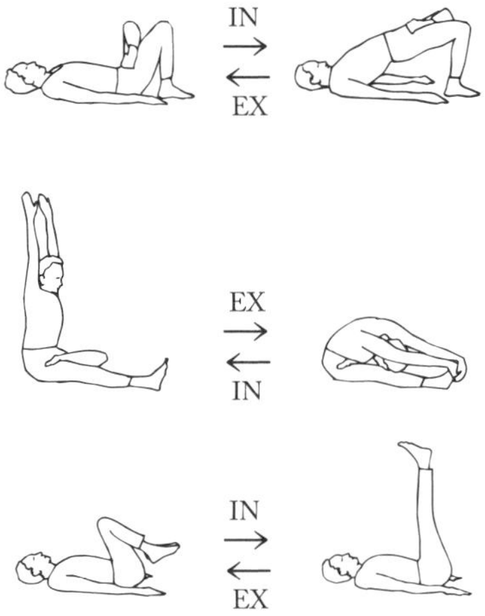
Prepare the body, breath, and mind to sit in the posture for pranayama practice.	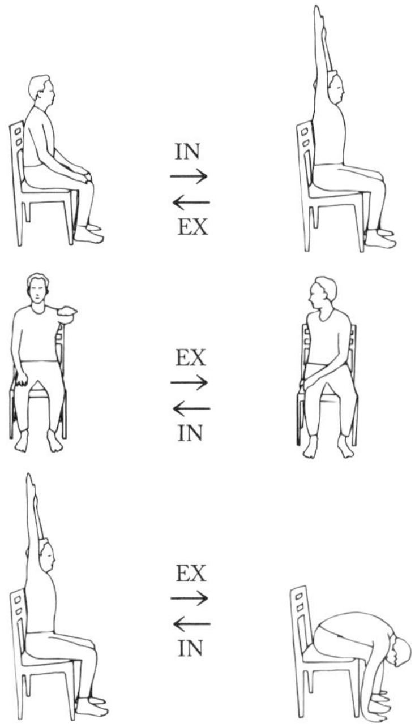	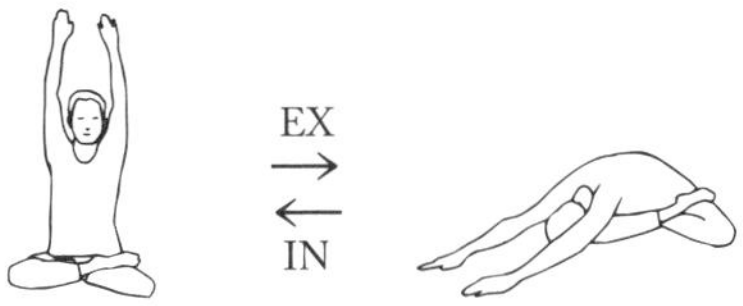
Rest and begin.	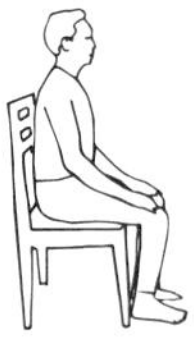	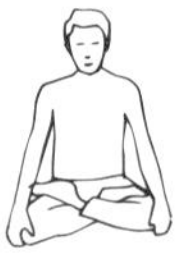

Fig. 6.4. Two examples illustrating the steps involved in preparing for pranayama.

unwise to load our stomach with food when elimination is incomplete, it is unwise to emphasize inhalation at the expense of exhalation. The quality of exhalation is a very important factor to be considered in determining the length and depth of inhalation. That is, the length or depth of inhalation should not be emphasized to the extent that the smoothness of exhalation is compromised. Increasing the length and smoothness of exhalation through appropriate practice should automatically lead to deeper and longer inhalation. Forcing inhalation increases rajas in the mind.

Retention after inhalation. Retention of air, or holding the breath after inhalation, can be considered a continuation of inhalation. Indeed, holding after inhalation is like holding on to inhalation. It is not possible to extend the length of exhalation or inhalation beyond a certain point, but holding after inhalation or exhalation allows us to extend their physical and psychological effects. Holding the breath after inhalation comes naturally to most people, since mental tension makes us do just this.

Suspension after exhalation. Suspension after exhalation is like fasting. We use the word *suspension* rather than *holding* because it implies a mental attitude of keeping things away rather than holding on to them. Suspension should not be extended to the point where the succeeding inhalation is rapid or forced. The limit of suspension is usually linked to the length of exhalation.

Inhalation-exhalation relationship. Inhalation and exhalation are the two main components of the breathing cycle. Although they have different characteristics, they are not opposing forces but complementary ones. Breathing is a continuous, cyclical movement. Neither inhalation nor exhalation can be completely stopped. We can only increase the duration of their presence or absence by extending any one of the components of the breathing cycle. The presence of one (inhalation or exhalation) implies the temporary absence of the other. When we exhale, there is an absence of inhalation during that period, and vice versa. When we increase the presence of one, we are automatically increasing the absence of the other.

Inhalation can be completed quickly, whereas exhalation cannot. For example, we can inhale fully in as little as three seconds, whereas it is not possible to exhale completely in the same time, unless it is forced. During inhalation, air goes in quickly, whereas during exhalation the air is not let out quickly. Inhalation is more active and exhalation more passive.

Why use ratios? The components of the breathing cycle have distinct effects on the body and the mind. It is possible to alter their lengths, varying the ratio between them, in order to bring about desired changes in the body and mind. For example, extended exhalation brings about a feeling of relaxation. Therefore, to relax, we can make the length of exhalation twice that of inhalation (a ratio of 1:0:2:0; that is: inhalation/holding after inhalation/

exhalation/suspension after exhalation). Similarly, to become more active or energized, we can make the length of inhalation equal to that of exhalation (a ratio of 1:0:1:0).

If all the components are of equal length, the pranayama is called *sama-vrtti-pranayama* and if unequal, *vishama-vrtti-pranayama*. The word *sama* means "equal," and *vishama* means "unequal." *Vrtti* means "movement." For example, a ratio of 1:1:1:1 constitutes sama-vrtti-pranayama, while any other ratio, such as 1:4:2:1, is vishama-vrtti-pranayama.

The ratio that you choose will depend upon your purpose. For example, for the purpose of calming down or relaxation, you could use 3 seconds for inhalation and 6 seconds for exhalation if you have shortness of breath. If you are a fit person, you could use 8 seconds for inhalation and 16 seconds for exhalation and repeat this for, say, 16 breaths. Similarly, if you have shortness of breath but want to be more active, you could use a ratio of 5:0:5:0. If you are fit and want to be more active, try using 12:0:12:0.

Pranayama involves conscious regulation of two complementary forces—the inhalation and the exhalation—with a specific purpose in mind. You must always take into account the quality of your breath and the present state of your mind. Ratios must not be fixed or unvarying. Alter them during a practice session if necessary. Do not fix a ratio and force your breath. This can lead to an imbalance in the breath, just as fixing a form and forcing the body in asana practice can cause an imbalance in the body. For instance, indis-criminate retention of the breath can lead to tremors and psychological tension.

Lengthening the inhalation or exhalation should not be done at the expense of uniformity; there should be steadiness or uniformity (dirgha) and smoothness or fineness (sukshma). The steadiness and smoothness of the breath over a number of cycles are key. Dirgha and sukshma should be maintained on inhalation as well as exhalation. If we try to force the breathing pattern into a ratio that is inappropriate at that particular time—perhaps propelled by our ego into "achieving" that ratio, or simply due to a lack of knowledge, awareness, or skill—we will sacrifice sukshma, or smoothness of breath. It is wise to remember that the breath cannot be forced like the body. The breath is under our control only to a limited extent. Breathing is considered one of the natural urges (*vega*s) in Ayurveda. Forcing the breath can disturb our physical and mental functions. That is why texts such as the *Hatha-Yoga-Pradipika* caution us against an improper pranayama practice. In order to maintain a proper relationship between inhalation and exhalation, we have to consider the following:

1. One should not disturb the other. Both should be long, uniform, and deep.
2. Inhalation and exhalation should complement and promote each other when repeated over a number of cycles.
3. The uniformity, depth, and fineness of the breath (sukshma), not merely its length, must be the basis for determining the ratio. There should be absence of fluctuation.

4. The type of pranayama must be chosen based on your needs. Observe the condition of your throat, nostrils, and so on. The methodology of breathing chosen should help to maintain uniformity, depth, and length. Proper techniques can make the exhalation and inhalation smoother.

Desha, Kala, and Samkhya

Desha means "place." In this context, it is the place where the mind is focused. *Kala* means "time," referring to the duration of the components of the breathing cycle. *Samkhya* means "number" and refers to the number of cycles of breathing to be done. Desha, kala, and samkhya are interrelated. They are also related to the different components of the breath. The interconnection between all these factors has to be understood clearly and applied appropriately to make the breath long and steady (dirgha) and smooth and subtle (sukshma).

Dirgha and sukshma are interrelated characteristics: Dirgha is long and sukshma is deep. Trees that are tall have deep roots. The breath should be not only long but also deep. Depth refers to absence of mental fluctuation; the deeper we dive into the sea, the fewer the waves. It is worth noting that in the sutra on dirgha and sukshma (*Yoga-Sutras* 2.50) the word *vrtti*, or "movement" is used, as in the definition of yoga (*Yoga-Sutras* 1.2). This emphasizes the importance of the connection between the movement of the breath and that of the mind. Therefore, the emphasis should be on how we link our mind and breath so that we can dive deep into ourselves during the practice of pranayama.

Mantra in Pranayama

The ancient texts spoke about pranayama being practiced with mantra, especially the *gayatri*-mantra. (The concept of mantra has been explained in my book *Yoga for Body, Breath, and Mind*). Mantra is used as a unit for measuring the length of breath. The ratio suggested was 1:1:1:0 using the gayatri-mantra. It is also common to use a short mantra like AUM or RAM. Pranayama when done with mantra is called *sa-mantraka* or *sa-garbha* ("with seed"). The seed here is the mantra, which grows to fruition as the practice proceeds. Pranayama without use of mantra is called *a-mantraka* or *a-garbha* ("without seed").

THE RESULTS OF PRANAYAMA

We can say that to practice pranayama we choose a suitable posture and then modify the pattern of breathing. We also take into account desha, kala, and samkhya so that the breath has the qualities of dirgha and sukshma.

According to the *Yoga-Sutras*, as a result of practicing pranayama properly, there is removal of the covering of the light of the Seer (*Yoga-Sutras* 2.52) and the mind becomes fit for focus (*dharana*) (2.53).

The same idea has been expressed

differently in other texts like the *Hatha-Yoga-Pradipika* and *Yoga-Yajnavalkya,* with prana rather than the mind as the focus. For example, the *Hatha-Yoga-Pradipika* states that the nadis are cleansed (*Hatha-Yoga-Pradipika* 2.6) and the prana is focused and moves up the *sushumna.*

Prana flows in the body through innumerable subtle channels or conduits called nadis. Obstruction of the flow of prana in the nadis results in disease. Restoration of health involves the cleansing of the nadis. This allows prana to resume its normal flow. The focusing of the prana happens automatically as the mind becomes quieter during the practice of pranayama. The removal of the covering of the light of the Seer will result from the cleansing of the nadis.

The *Hatha-Yoga-Pradipika* and other texts also give details about the use of *bandha*s and *mudra*s in the practice of pranayama. We also find references in the texts to the concept of *agni,* which occupies a central role in Ayurveda. Agni is the metabolic "fire," the heat or energy responsible for the transformation of food into the seven *dhatu*s (body tissues), each one being derived from its predecessor. Texts such as the *Hatha-Yoga-Pradipika* make extensive use of the theory of Ayurveda to explain the effects of pranayama practice, and hence we find the use of not only the term *agni,* but also several other Ayurvedic terms such as Vata, Pitta, and Kapha and the names of many diseases.

UNDERSTANDING PRANA IN YOGA

Prana and the mind can be considered two aspects of the power (shakti) of the Seer. The mind is the manifestation of the ability of the Seer to cognize (*jnana-shakti*), while the prana is the energy of the Seer that drives this process (*kriya-shakti*). They are deeply and intricately linked. When the mind is disturbed, the flow of prana is disturbed, which in turn disturbs the flow of the breath and the functioning of the body (*Yoga-Sutras* 1.31). Asana and pranayama make use of this connection by using the body and the breath to reduce disturbance in the mind. Consequently, the disturbance in the flow of prana is also reduced.

In other yoga texts, such as the *Hatha-Yoga-Pradipika,* this is referred to as the focusing of the prana from the *ida* and *pingala* into the sushumna. The conversion of a disturbed mind to a focused one is equivalent to the conversion of the prana from a scattered to a focused state. It is a gradual process requiring patient, sustained effort.

Two important channels, or nadis, in which prana flows in the body are the ida and pingala. The terminal points of these two nadis are the nostrils. The pingala (right side) is related to the sun, representing heat, and the ida (left side) is related to the moon, representing cold. Thus, breathing through the left nostril and breathing through the right nostril are said to have different effects on the internal balance of the system.

Mudras and Bandhas

Mudra means "seal." In texts such as the *Hatha-Yoga-Pradipika*, it is suggested that certain practices that focus the mind can center the prana. These are termed mudras. The practice of mudras helps to prevent the scattering of prana and thus aids in achieving focus of the mind. For example, in *shan-mukhi-mudra*, we close the ears, eyes, and mouth with our fingers and thumbs. This temporarily prevents the outward movement of the senses. In *cin-mudra*, we place the forefinger on the thumb. In *anjali-mudra*, the hands are placed together like a lotus flower.

In the *Hatha-Yoga-Pradipika* (3.77–82), the headstand, shoulder stand, and other related inverted positions are classified under *viparita-karani*, one of the ten mudras. Other texts such as the *Shiva-Samhita* (4.45–47) and *Gheranda-Samhita* (3.33–36) also classify headstand as one of the mudras.

Bandhas are also grouped with mudras, as they serve the same purpose. The word *bandha* means "to bind" or "to lock." Bandhas include certain physical practices involving muscular contractions, designed to block or seal off certain areas of the body and thus redirect the flow of prana. The three important bandhas used in the practice of pranayama are *mula-bandha, uddiyana-bandha*, and *jalandhara-bandha*. An important use of the practice of bandhas is to enhance the functioning of agni. This happens more as a result of the use of appropriate breathing than from body work. For

example, in headstand we can practice *mula-bandha* and *uddiyana-bandha*, but for this practice to be truly effective, long and deep breathing is essential. Another bandha sometimes used in pranayama is *jihva-bandha*. Here the tongue is rolled back so that the tip touches the back of the palate.

The practice of jalandhara-bandha. The practice of *jalandhara-bandha* involves straightening the spine, relaxing the abdomen, slightly pulling the head back, and then lowering the head. The chest must rise to meet the chin; the head must not be forced down. When done properly, *jalandhara-bandha* helps in doing *mula-bandha*. Breath plays a vital role in the practice of the bandhas. Therefore, lengthening and controlling the breath in asana practice is essential before attempting to do *jalandhara-bandha*. In *jalandhara-bandha*, the upper part of the upper back is rounded and the neck is slightly hyperextended. Therefore, it must be practiced only if there is sufficient strength and flexibility in the neck and back. Postures like *dvipadapitham* help to prepare for the practice of *jalandhara-bandha*.

The practice of mula-bandha. The practice of *mula-bandha* involves contraction of the lower abdomen below the navel. Extended exhalation involves contraction of the abdominal muscles, and thus performing *mula-bandha* in suspension after exhalation allows one to use the natural link between muscular work and the breathing process. Inverted positions such as headstand and shoulder stand also facilitate the performance of *mula-bandha*. According to classical yoga texts like the *Hatha-Yoga-Pradipika, mula-bandha* is to be maintained throughout the practice of pranayama. This can be done effectively only if inhalation starts in the chest. That is, inhaling is done following the chest-to-abdomen method and not vice versa. *Asvini-mudra* should not be confused with *mula-bandha*. The former involves conscious contraction of the external anal sphincter.

The practice of uddiyana-bandha. The practice of *uddiyana-bandha* and *mula-bandha* are related. *Uddiyana-bandha* involves contraction of the upper abdomen as well, elevating the navel and drawing it inward.

Both *uddiyana-bandha* and *mula-bandha* are not to be attempted on inhalation and in back bends. They should be done after exhalation, slowly, with awareness, and with *jalandhara-bandha*.

Once *jalandhara-bandha* and *mula-bandha* are assumed in the practice of pranayama, they are to be maintained throughout, while *uddiyana-bandha* is to be done on suspension after exhalation and released before inhalation. Again, the purpose of the bandhas is to prevent the prana from moving upward and the apana from moving downward so that both are retained. *Jalandhara-bandha* helps to arrest the upward movement of the prana, and *mula-bandha* the downward movement of apana. Pranayama, as we have said, can be considered a process of balancing prana and apana, thus the importance of maintaining these two bandhas throughout pranayama practice.

Improper practice of the bandhas can result in many health problems. In most cases, similar benefits can be achieved by safer and better means like the use of sound.

Regulation of the Breath

The flow of the breath can be regulated at the throat or at the nostrils. Table 6.3 summarizes the breathing techniques of the various pranayama practices outlined in the classical yoga texts.

Regulation at the throat. We can regulate the flow of breath by constricting the throat (the glottis). Such breathing is called *ujjayi*, meaning "that which helps to gain mastery over the chest." This constriction of the throat creates a sound as the air flows past; this sound can be used as an indicator of the smoothness of the flow of the breath and provides feedback to help us enhance the regulation of its flow. Jalandhara-bandha can help in this process.

Regulation at the nostrils. Regulation of the flow of breath at the nostrils involves closing one nostril fully and the other partially. It is best to allow the fingers to rest on the nostrils, just below the bridge of the nose, not close to the tip. Both inhalation and exhalation can be controlled in this manner. During exhalation, it is vital to ensure that there is no back pressure. The primary method for regulating the breath is controlling diaphragmatic movement. This is achieved through the

TABLE 6.3. **Various types of pranayama, as mentioned in classical yoga texts.**

	Pranayama	Inhalation	Exhalation	Variations
1.	*Anuloma-ujjayi*	Throat	Alternate nostrils	Exhale - left nostril Exhale - right nostril
2.	*Viloma-ujjayi*	Alternate nostrils	Throat	
3.	*Pratiloma-ujjayi*	Throat Left nostril Throat Right nostril	Left nostril Throat Right nostril Throat	1 round consists of 4 breaths
4.	*Shitali*	Mouth with folded tongue	Throat or 1 nostril	Exhale - throat Exhale - left nostril Exhale - right nostril
5.	*Sitkari*	Mouth with tongue flat between slightly opened teeth	Throat or 1 nostril	Exhale - throat Exhale - left nostril Exhale - right nostril
6.	*Nadishodhana*	Left nostril Right nostril	Right nostril Left nostril	1 round consists of 2 breaths alternating: L in, R out, R in, L out
7.	*Suryabhedana*	Right nostril	Left nostril	
8.	*Chandrabhedana*	Left nostril	Right nostril	
9.	*Kapalabhati*	Both nostrils, stomach forward	Both nostrils, stomach in	Fast abdominal breathing. Variations of exhalation and inhalation possible.
10.	*Bhastrika*	Left nostril Right nostril	Left nostril Right nostril	Fast abdominal breathing. Variations of exhalation and inhalation possible.
11.	*Murcha*	Deep	Long	Emphasis on extended exhalation.
12.	*Plavini*	Quick inhalation and long hold after inhalation	Free	Emphasis on holding after inhalation.

proper application of the methodology of breathing (chest to abdomen on inhalation and abdomen to chest on exhalation). The nostrils are a secondary point of control. If we cannot regulate the breath through diaphragmatic movement and keep the breath smooth, long, and steady, then we will get a feeling that the breath wants to force itself out. This is what is meant by back pressure.

Breathing through both nostrils. We can try to extend exhalation or inhalation as we breathe normally through both nostrils, through control at the diaphragm alone. However, such extension of the breath is limited.

Inhalation through the mouth. Inhalation through the mouth is done in certain types of pranayama like shitali and sit-kari. Here too, extension of inhalation is achieved mainly through control at the diaphragm.

PRANAYAMA FOR THERAPY

Classical yoga texts explain how various types of pranayama can be linked to the doshas and to qualities of heat and cold. To use pranayama as a therapeutic tool, we need to understand these connections clearly. Although the details are not within the scope of this chapter, below is a brief outline of the steps to be followed in designing a pranayama practice for therapeutic purposes:

- Assess the person's constitution.
- Determine which dosha is out of balance

based on the disease and which dosha is out of balance in the person.
- Select the type of pranayama.
- Determine the appropriate ratio to be followed, taking into account both the person and the problem.
- Decide on the mental focus for the person.
- Choose the appropriate posture for practicing pranayama.
- Define the necessary preparatory steps for both the posture and the breath.
- Teach the pranayama.

OBSERVATION, SEQUENCING, AND PERSONALIZATION IN PRANAYAMA

We have explained in detail how observation, sequencing, and personalization form the core steps in designing an asana practice. All three are equally applicable in pranayama as well, and the approach is similar but will not be explained in detail here. We present below an idea of how this approach should be applied to pranayama.

Observing

- Observe the body to choose the right posture for pranayama. Consider whether the person is fit or unwell.
- Observe the length and smoothness of each component of the breath and the methodology of breathing. This will help you decide on an appropriate ratio.
- Observe the behavior and inquire about

the background of the person to decide what form of mental focus will be most suitable for that person—what can he or she relate to?

Sequencing

Prepare the person to do the ratio over a period of time. For example, start with a ratio of 6:0:12:0 and successively introduce ratios of 6:0:12:6, 6:6:12:6, and finally, 6:12:12:6. This has to be done over several practice sequences.

Personalizing

- Use supports to make the posture in which the person does pranayama more stable and comfortable.
- Use sound in addition to the pranayama.
- Modify the ratio, number of cycles, and other components of the pranayama to suit the person.

Please see appendix B for questions related to the practice of pranayama.

PART THREE

Yoga and Ayurveda as Therapy

Part three discusses yoga and Ayurveda in the context of therapy. Chapter 7 outlines some of the principles of yoga and Ayurveda that can be used therapeutically. Chapter 8 uses case studies to illustrate how these principles can be applied in particular therapeutic situations. In the case studies that involve a structural problem, we emphasize the application of yoga principles. In cases involving a functional problem, we emphasize the use of Ayurveda as the principal therapy.

The content of part three will be especially useful for yoga teachers and for therapists who are using yoga and Ayurveda, but all yoga practitioners will find this material helpful. Many common complaints that affect almost everyone at some point—back pain, headache, constipation, insomnia, and menstrual problems—are considered here. The case studies provide information that you can use to find a solution for these problems.

In chapter 1, we listed six factors that can be used to maintain and restore balance in our body and mind: diet, environment, lifestyle, body work (asanas), breathing techniques (pranayama), and our thoughts and emotions. We have discussed what asana and pranayama are, described their important features, and explained many principles regarding how they should be done in order to maintain health. Mostly, these principles apply in therapeutic situations as well. Part three addresses the two other major factors—diet and mental techniques—outlining the salient features of Ayurvedic dietetics and explaining the key role of the mind in effecting positive change.

The Practice of Yoga and Ayurveda Therapy

7

WHAT IS therapy? We use the word *therapy* in place of what yoga and Ayurveda call *cikitsa*, a Sanskrit word meaning "to oppose or act against disease." Caraka, the author of the most respected treatise on Ayurveda, defines disease as *duhkha*. Duhkha is a feeling of not being at ease, just as the word *dis-ease* itself implies this state of mind. Duhkha is a feeling of mental constriction, of circumstances being unfavorable to us. It could manifest in many ways, from anger to depression. The opposite is the feeling of mental expansion, the lightness and freedom that we feel when circumstances are, in our judgment, favorable to us (*sukha* in Sanskrit). All of us are aware of both these states of mind. We continually oscillate between them throughout our lives. All experiences, in the present or the past, have the potential to

bring about these feelings of expansion and constriction in our mental space, though the intensity varies depending on the experience.

In terms of the three gunas, the state of mind in which sattva predominates is the one in which we have the least duhkha. The contentment and fulfillment that characterize sattva naturally imply an absence of duhkha.

It is obvious that all of us continually strive to minimize the duhkha in our lives. Undeniably, our ultimate goal is to remove all duhkha—to remain at ease always, irrespective of any external circumstances, even those of our own body. Being at ease is a state of mind, not of the body. The *Yoga-Sutras* say precisely this. From their point of view, all of us, even those we would normally consider healthy, are in need of cikitsa, or therapy, because none of us is ever completely free from duhkha, or dis-ease. The *Yoga-Sutras* say that it is possible to always remain in a state of sattva—to be without duhkha at all—and they describe the steps to be taken to move toward this goal.

In our present state, the connection between our mind and body runs deep. Our state of mind is inextricably linked to that of our body. Disturbance of body structure or function is reflected as a lack of ease in our mind. We are incapable of being mentally at ease in the face of physical illness. Consequently, our mental well-being rests on the foundation of physical well-being. Any approach to relieve dis-ease must take into account this connection between the body and mind. Therefore, Ayurveda deals first with the prevention and treatment of physical illness and then moves to the consideration of mental wellness. Similarly, the practice of yoga for achieving mental freedom requires us to be physically healthy. Therefore, the *Yoga-Sutras* tell us that the practice of the various disciplines outlined in the eight limbs of yoga must not be at the expense of the body: It must not disturb our physical health.

That is, we need to ensure that our body and mind function in a balanced manner before we look toward higher goals. To repeat what was said in chapter 1: Just like any other object in this world, our body has various qualities and functions. Health requires balanced expression of the body's qualities and functions.

Therapy consists of restoring balance in these qualities and functions. In other words, therapy involves instituting measures to resolve the disruption in function or return the expression of body qualities to their normal, balanced level. But this raises a question: What constitutes a "balance" of qualities and functions in our body? What should we consider imbalance?

AYURVEDIC CONSTITUTION

What is the normal range within which the qualities and functions in our body should be expressed? Beyond what limits would we consider a quality or function of the body to be abnormal or to require therapy? One answer is that abnormality is subjective. This is true in one sense. But, objectively, normality is the range within which the majority of the population falls. This varies for any particular quality or function. The range of normality is clear when the criterion is easily quantifiable, such as heart rate or daily water intake. One person may drink six glasses of water a day, while another may drink ten. Both are normal. But consuming thirty glasses of water every day probably indicates some abnormality or disturbance in bodily function.

Ayurveda defines normality according to the concepts of specificity and commonality. Any object belongs to a class of objects, in which the members share certain common qualities. In fact, one or more of these common qualities are the basis for placing these objects together in one category. This is the commonality that spans these objects. Yet each object differs from the others by small variations in these qualities or by the presence of some other qualities. These constitute the specificity in each object. As humans, we have several qualities—structural, physiological, and psychological—that are common to us all. Yet each of these qualities varies to some extent in each of us. This is what makes each of us unique.

When variations in our body qualities are within certain limits, they differentiate us from one another but do not displace us from the category of normality and health. When any such variation is so large that it results in a marked change in structure or function, we consider it abnormal and a sign of ill health. For example, adult human beings range in height from around four feet to seven feet. We do not find adult human beings one foot or twelve feet tall. This approximate range of height comprises all of us. Yet each of us has our own exact height within this range. This is the specificity or individuality in us. The farther a person's height is from this common range, the greater the chance of its being a cause or result of ill health.

The Concept of Prakriti

A variation in any bodily or mental quality, if not large enough to be a cause or manifestation of ill health, is simply part of our normal or constitutional makeup, known as *prakriti* in Ayurveda. Since we have already classified body qualities and functions under three groups—the three doshas—we can also classify variations in them as an increase or decrease in one or more of the doshas. In this way, constitution can be expressed in terms of

the doshas. To do this properly, however, we need to be sure that the variation in the quality is not temporary. We need to know the relative importance of conflicting variations—because, as we noted in chapter 1, the three doshas share both similar and opposing qualities.

Inherent Tendencies toward Ill Health

We can then say that Ayurveda defines our health by reference to the unique imbalance in the qualities and functions of our body. As a result, inherent variations in those qualities and functions can indicate where our tendencies toward imbalances are greatest. A person may have skin that tends to dry relatively easily. Dryness is a quality of Vata. Right now, this may not be a cause of disease; the person may be healthy. But the potential always exists for this to become a problem, more so than in a person who has inherently oily skin.

The reason for assessing your constitution is to learn where these tendencies toward imbalance are greatest in you. Knowing this, you can be careful not to aggravate the imbalances already in your body.

FOOD: THE KEY CONNECTION

Among the many ways that the external world influences our body, food is the most important. Through food, a part of our environment becomes part of our body every day. Therefore, Ayurveda, which deals mainly with maintaining and restoring balance in our body, places utmost importance on the food we eat.

Appropriate Food

Food nourishes our body by becoming a part of it. It is the most direct connection between the qualities in the environment and those in our body—a physical factor that directly affects the balance in our body from within. Therefore, we cannot ignore the possible role of food in any functional problem in the body. In the face of an imbalanced, inappropriate diet, it is difficult to make significant progress in reducing disease or maintaining good health. In many cases, food can be a factor contributing to the sustenance or propagation of a disease, and changing the person's food habits will be a large part of the treatment.

Food as Medicine

Both food and medicine are substances that we consume. We usually take food regularly and in large quantities, whereas we consume medicines in small quantities and only when ill. Therefore, we usually view food as something that gives us energy and maintains our health, while we associate medicine with illness.

In Ayurveda, because the medicines suggested are mostly herbal, and because of the importance attached to food in maintaining and restoring health, the same basic rules of dietetics are applied to both food and medicines. In other words, food is considered to be medicine, only less potent.

Below we explore the connections between food and the qualities and functions in our body, and how food can be used to restore health and maintain balance in our body and mind.

THE AYURVEDIC APPROACH TO DIETETICS

For our health to be maintained, the qualities and functions of our body must be in balance. Therapy consists of restoring this balance. To do this using food, we need to know how various food items affect the qualities and functions in our body and how to use this knowledge to design a diet for a particular person.

We need to know how to link the qualities in food items to the changes they produce in the qualities of the body. Ayurveda explains this in two ways. The first is by the taste of the food item. Taste is something we can directly experience, but it is only a broad and variable indicator. The second method is by a direct reference to the changes that the food item produces in the body. This may be a description of the body qualities that the food item affects, or it may be more specific and related to a particular body system or disease.

Food qualities are not directly linked to their effect on the body, however. Although our body tissues are formed from food, we are structurally different from the food we eat. We may eat apples or drink milk, and they may affect the qualities in our body and functioning of our body systems in different ways, but they do not alter the fundamental nature of our body tissues. This is because food is transformed into our body tissues once it enters our body. That is, though food becomes part of our body, it is fundamentally transformed in the process.

Because of this transformation, the physical qualities in food itself are unrelated to those in our body. For example, our bones are hard, but eating hard foods will not increase bone density. Similarly, if we have dry skin, consuming more oil in our diet is not a direct way to address the problem. This is an oversimplification and an ineffective approach.

Since the physical qualities in the food are not a guide to their effect on the body, they are of limited relevance in maintaining health or providing therapy. When Ayurveda describes various qualities in food substances (hot, dry, cold, oily, heavy, and so on), this does not refer to the physical qualities of a particular food item but to its effect on our body.

For instance, when we describe a substance as dry, this means that it will increase the quality of dryness in the body. Such a substance can have, for example, a constipating effect. The food itself may or may not be physically dry; we may even drink it as a liquid preparation.

In the same way, substances that are said to be heating are not necessarily themselves hot, although they could be. Usually, they help to increase some aspects of body metabolism, which in turn can be expressed as increased heat. For instance, they can stimulate digestion or accelerate inflammatory processes, which may be useful or not, depending on the situation.

Heavy and light are qualities of food that describe the ease or difficulty with which they are digested. Food that can be digested and absorbed most easily by the body, in the least time and with minimum effort, are said to be light. Heavy food takes longer to be digested and absorbed. For example, porridge made from roasted rice is very light and more digestible than cooked rice. Many foods become more difficult to digest when deep-fried in oil.

Food may be heavier or lighter relative to the state of one's digestion. A fit thirty-year-old man who is used to vigorous exercise may be able to digest a large meal quite easily. A sedentary sixty-year-old man, however, may find similar food much more difficult to digest.

Of the twenty body qualities listed in figure 1.2 (see page 8), three pairs are the most important, especially when considering the effect of food items on the body. They are hot and cold, dry and oily, and light and heavy. Again, each of these represents a food item's effect on the body, not the nature of the food item itself.

These qualities may be understood in terms of the presence of one indicating the absence of its opposite. For instance, cold is absence of heat, dryness is absence of oiliness or wetness, and lightness is absence of heaviness. In general, it is easier to use food to add to the qualities of the body rather than diminish them, because eating is itself a process of addition. Therefore, it is often easier to increase heat, oiliness, and heaviness than to remove them.

AGNI

In order to design an appropriate diet, whether the person is healthy or unwell, we need a clear understanding of the concept of agni.

Heat and Biological Transformation

Energy plays a role in most biological transformations. In all biological systems, some metabolic transformations require energy, and some others release energy. As a simple and easily observable example, consider an orange on a tree. When unripe, it tastes sour. As time passes, it ripens and comes to taste sweet. An apple is bitter as a seed, sour when unripe, and finally sweet when mature. These transformations require energy in the form of heat provided by the sun. The plant absorbs the energy of sunlight and uses it to power these transformations in the fruit. If we remove the fruit from the tree too early, it may rot instead of ripening.

Fire is the most obvious source of heat and energy in the world around us. When we heat food to cook it, it undergoes changes in color, texture, taste, and other qualities. Similarly, food, once eaten, is "cooked" inside our body. Its qualities are transformed in the process of digestion, absorption, distribution, and use by our body tissues.

Energy is required for most biological transformations, and the transformation of food inside our body is no exception. Ayurveda uses the concept of agni to explain the energy changes associated with these transformations. The word *agni* literally means "fire." The fundamental, defining quality of fire is not flame but the release of energy—the heat. Therefore, agni refers not to fire as such but to the energy responsible for and released by the transformations in our body, especially that of the food we eat.

Considering Agni in the Diet

Fire is necessary to burn fuel but is itself sustained by the fuel. Similarly, agni is responsible for the digestion, absorption, and utilization of food in our body, but it is itself sustained by the food we eat—or rather, by the energy released from the food we eat. Therefore, agni, or our body's metabolism, is deeply intertwined with the food we eat.

If agni is either deficient or excessive, the food we eat may not be digested and absorbed properly, and even if it is absorbed, it may not be used appropriately in the body. Designing a diet without considering the state of your agni is not correct, because the purpose of the food you eat is to nourish your body and keep it healthy—and agni is what makes this happen. If you ignore the state of your agni, the food you eat may be creating an imbalance in your body, even though your diet itself may appear to be balanced. Diabetes mellitus, for example, is a classic example of a condition in which the functioning of agni is impaired. A person with uncontrolled diabetes may eat well but will find it difficult to gain body mass because the food is not being used to nourish the body effectively.

Agni is not the only factor in treating disease, of course, but the proper functioning of agni is reflected in all body systems—from proper digestion to good energy and a feeling of mental lightness and clarity. Therefore, the status of one's agni is important as a general indicator of progress in treatment. The most direct indicator of the functioning of agni is naturally the functioning of the digestive system—not only the proper digestion and absorption of food but also the elimination of waste products.

THE ROLE OF TASTE

Among all the physical attributes of a food item, including its taste, texture, color, and shape, taste plays the greatest role in dictating our food habits. Taste is the most important physical quality of our food that we experience as food enters our body. Ayurveda focuses much attention on the taste of food and discusses in detail how the taste of a particular food can be used to judge the effect it will have on our body qualities.

The Six Tastes

Ayurveda lists six tastes: sweet, sour, salty, pungent, astringent, and bitter. Modern science acknowledges only four of these—sweet, sour, salty, and bitter—as real tastes. Pungent or hot, for example, is a sensation of irritation and burning rather than a taste as such. But all six of these sensations, whether or not they fall under the category of taste in modern terminology, can be perceived as we eat food and are useful in judging the effect a food can have on the body. This will become clearer as we explore the relationship of these tastes to various qualities and functions.

Taste and the Qualities in Food

The taste of a particular food indicates the relative predominance of qualities in it, especially of the six important qualities (hot, cold, dry, oily, heavy, and light). The association of taste with these six qualities is the primary basis underlying the connections we make between the six tastes and the five elements, and between the six tastes and the three doshas.

We can relate the five elements to the six tastes as listed in table 7.1. What this means is that a foodstuff with a particular taste is likely to increase in our body the qualities associated with the corresponding elements.

For example, the quality of heaviness is associated with earth and water. We know only too well that otherwise healthy people will put on weight if they eat too many sweets. Thus, the association between the sweet taste and the earth and water elements makes sense in terms of our own experience. Astringent substances are heavy and drying but not heating. We see this combination of qualities only in the combination of the elements earth and air. Similarly, pungent

TABLE 7.1. The relationship among the tastes, elements, and six important qualities.

TASTE	ELEMENTS	QUALITIES
Sweet	Earth, water	Oily, heavy, cold
Sour	Earth, fire	Oily, heavy, hot
Salty	Water, fire	Oily, light, hot
Pungent	Fire, air	Dry, light, hot
Bitter	Air, space	Dry, light, cold
Astringent	Air, earth	Dry, heavy, cold

substances increase body metabolism and heat and stimulate movement. These qualities are found only in two elements taken together—fire and air. The other element/taste connections can be understood in a similar fashion. As you can see, the basis of these connections is the similarity in distribution of qualities—primarily of the six important ones (hot, cold, dry, oily, heavy, and light)—among the five elements and the six tastes. Similarly, we can posit a relationship between the tastes and an increase or decrease in the three doshas as well (table 7.2).

The Three Postdigestive Tastes

The relationship between the tastes and the doshas is somewhat complex, as you can see from table 7.2. A food with a particular taste will affect the qualities of more than one

TABLE 7.2. The relative predominance of the six important qualities in foodstuffs based on their taste.

TASTE	VATA	PITTA	KAPHA
Sweet	⬇	⬇	⬇
Sour	⬇	⬇	⬇
Salty	⬇	⬇	⬇
Pungent	⬆	⬆	⬆
Bitter	⬆	⬆	⬆
Astringent	⬆	⬆	⬆

dosha. To make this relationship more simple, Ayurveda proposes the concept of *vipaka,* which is the change the tastes undergo after contact with agni (that is, after digestion). The six tastes can be reduced to three to relate them more easily to the three doshas, and as a general rule, this is done as follows:

- Sweet and salty become sweet (Kapha).
- Sour remains sour (Pitta).
- Pungent, bitter, and astringent become pungent (Vata).

Apart from simplifying the connection of the tastes to the doshas, this concept is also used to explain how some foodstuffs have a particular taste but increase the qualities related to some other taste. For some of these foods, it is suggested, the postdigestive taste is different from the original taste. For example, many legumes are sweet in taste (Kapha), but they increase some of the qualities associated with Vata, so they are said to have a pungent postdigestive taste.

Potency: Heating or Cooling

Of the six important qualities, Ayurveda designates two—hot and cold—as the most important. This is because heat is related to the functioning of agni in the body, which is essential for life. A disturbance in heat or cold, from the Ayurvedic standpoint, may indicate a disorder of body metabolism that can be reflected in any of the body systems.

Also, the way in which the effects of particular foods are expressed in the body is related to whether they are heating or cooling. In some situations, we may have a choice between heating and cooling substances that may achieve a similar effect. For example, both heating and cooling substances can be drying, but they act differently. If a person has a tendency toward loose stools, foods with mild drying (or constipating) action can be useful to contain this tendency. Ayurveda suggests both heating and cooling foods and medicines that have this effect. We will have to choose between them based on other associated symptoms and factors, including the person's digestive capability, energy level, and body constitution.

OTHER QUALITIES AND FUNCTIONS OF FOOD

Apart from taste, postdigestive taste, potency, and the important qualities of food items (mainly the twenty listed in figure 1.2), Ayurveda also describes various other properties of specific foods. These properties are usually the effect these foods have on specific body functions or systems. Some of these effects are related to the qualities of the food, but others cannot be explained on the basis of the qualities alone. For example, various foods are described as purgative, increasing appetite, nourishing, bad for the skin, and so on.

These are pointers to an assortment of specific uses of various foodstuffs and herbs. Many medicinal combinations of herbs suggested in Ayurveda usually include one or two herbs with such specific actions on the disease process or body system. Such knowledge is also useful in avoiding some foods in certain conditions. Thus this knowledge becomes significant in designing the best treatment for various imbalances.

DESIGNING A DIET

When designing a diet using the principles of Ayurveda, the most important question to be answered is: For whom?

Several characteristics of the person need to be considered, the first among them being whether the person is healthy or unwell. If the person is suffering from some specific imbalance, then the diet can be designed with the focus on correcting that imbalance. You can see this in the case studies presented in chapter 8.

However, many of us do not have specific health problems at any given moment, and therefore, the focus of our diet could be difficult to define. The idea of using prakriti, or constitution, as the main factor on which to base a diet is commonly proposed as an answer to this problem. Many books have been written detailing how to determine your prakriti and design your diet according to it. The idea has its merits, but that is not the approach of this book, and you will soon see why.

Considering Prakriti

What is the basis for using prakriti to recommend a certain diet? As we have discussed, a person's prakriti describes his or her inherent tendencies toward imbalance, and therefore it can point to the nature of future disease. In designing a diet based on prakriti, we are trying to use diet to prevent our inherent imbalances from increasing to the point where they result in disease. But prakriti is only a broad classification of body types, based on the natural variation in qualities or functions from person to person. Therefore, a truly personalized diet is not actually based on prakriti but on the specific nature of the imbalances in that person.

That is, to design a personalized diet, it is not sufficient to know that your prakriti is Vata, Pitta, Kapha, or, more confusing, some combination of these. More important is the knowledge of what qualities and functions are not in balance in your system. Your diet must be designed to address these specific imbalances. For example, dry skin; a thin, tall, bony body frame; or hard stools and infrequent bowel movement can each contribute to the classification of a person as belonging to Vata prakriti. But the diets we would design to minimize the potential of each of these imbalances to manifest as disease will differ in some significant aspects. There certainly are people whom we would broadly classify as a Vata prakriti who have regular and free bowel movement. It is obvious that a diet designed to increase the bulk or softness of stools would be pointless for such a person. Other factors—such as a significant potential to develop stiffness, joint pain, and even conditions like osteoarthritis—may be the reason we place someone in the category of Vata prakriti. The person's diet, lifestyle, and exercise should all be oriented toward keeping this tendency in check.

To repeat, a simple classification of people under three broad categories—as Vata, Pitta, or Kapha—or even as combinations of these three is not the best basis for a comprehensive, personalized diet plan. Your diet must be tailored to your individual needs, based on the specific imbalances in the qualities and functions of your body. In fact, this is absolutely true of all six factors we have listed as ways of achieving better health: diet, lifestyle, environment, asana, pranayama, and mental changes. This is why classical texts on Ayurveda do not attach any special importance to prakriti when suggesting guidelines for a balanced diet. In fact, the most significant guideline that these texts suggest is to include food items with all six tastes in our diet.

Matching Food to the Agni

Food items that are heavy or difficult to digest can be made light or easy to digest by cooking. The plants, fruits, and vegetables that we eat have, in a way, already been cooked by exposure to the heat of the sun. During the process of cooking, heat brings about a transformation of the food product. Even so, while fruits can generally be eaten raw, other plant parts like leaves, stems, roots, and tubers should be cooked before we eat them. Similarly, meat should be cooked, since the human body is not designed to eat or digest raw meat.

What this means is that food should be prepared so that it matches the person's agni, or metabolism. This is analogous to personalizing asanas. As we saw, if a person has a history of back pain, we must modify the movements in his asana practice to start from where he is and then gradually strengthen his back. Similarly, if a person's agni is weak, we need to modify her food to suit her agni and gradually build up her agni, using appropriate herbs if needed.

This principle of modifying food items to suit the agni is of central importance in Ayurvedic theory. Cooking is an important method of altering the heaviness or lightness of food so that it is made more acceptable to an individual's agni. For example, the agni is not very strong in an infant, but it becomes very active during adulthood and finally is less active in old age. Therefore, we must match the food product to suit the agni as the person ages or as his or her health condition changes. For example, if an old person is ill and wants to eat an apple, it may be best to bake the apple and remove the skin first. In the case of a young person who is sick, the apple may be eaten raw without the skin. This is similar to modifying asanas to optimize them for the person, choosing a suitable ratio of breathing in pranayama, or suggesting a personalized method of meditation.

The Role of the Mind

We know that the world around us is the source of myriad stimuli: colors and shapes, sounds, tastes, smells, and textures. We perceive these properties of objects through our senses: vision, hearing, taste, smell, and touch.

The instruments that make such perception possible are our sense organs: eyes, ears, tongue, nose, and skin. They convey these sensations to the mind. Based on these sensations and the memory of past experiences stored in it, the mind continuously generates thoughts and feelings. These thoughts and feelings are the basis for our actions. That is, the mind receives input about the world around us through our senses and then commands our body to act. The body is the vehicle that translates the thoughts of the mind into physical action. All actions stem from thoughts in the mind. In a way, thought is itself action in mind. Finally, our actions themselves are usually directed toward feeding a particular input to the senses. This then forms a complete cycle of sensory input, mental processing, and thought or action usually directed toward the attainment or avoidance of further sensory input of some sort.

This cycle operates ceaselessly in all of us, without respite, all through our waking hours. The mind is the central player in this cycle, as it determines what action to take, which in turn determines what sensations will be available to our senses. Therefore, both our senses and the body are under the control of the mind.

To illustrate with an example, let us say there is an apple on a table in my kitchen. When I enter the kitchen and happen to look at the apple, the apple's form and color are grasped by my eyes and sent to my mind. My mind now draws upon its data bank—the memory of past experiences—and recalls that apples (or rather, objects with that particular form and color) have tasted sweet in the past. Since sweet tastes are pleasurable to most of us, my mind has built within it a strong association of pleasure with eating the apple. This prompts the emergence of the next line of thought, now directed toward obtaining the apple. Once the thought that I should eat the apple has entered my mind, it orders my body to do what is required. Therefore, I reach for the apple with my hand, place it in my mouth, and bite it. The apple tastes sweet, and therefore the association of pleasure with the apple is further reinforced.

In this entire cycle, the mind plays the key role. The mere presence of the apple, or even the effect of its form and color on my eyes, means nothing to me unless my mind takes notice of it. Further, though my mind may acknowledge the information that my eyes provide about the existence of the apple, the decision as to whether to act on it, and what the nature of the action should be, is again made only by the mind.

Upon reflection, we can see that our entire lives function within this cycle. It is nothing new to us. We can easily see this happening all the time. In a way, we could say that this cycle is simply an expression of our processing loop! The mind receives input through the senses. It then processes it and directs the body to deliver the appropriate output as actions.

An impairment in the functioning of any one of the components in this cycle, or in the connections between them, is a cause for disorder or disease. All components of this loop must function as they should, with their connections intact, if our lives are to proceed smoothly. For example, if my eyes are unable to see the apple in daylight, there is something wrong with them. We could also express this as a disorder in the connection between the sense organ (the eye) and the sense object (the form and color of the apple). Similarly, it is obvious that the inability or diminished ability to perceive any of the other modalities of sensation also constitutes a disability or disease.

If my eyes are fine but my mind is unable to recall the details about apples I have eaten in the past, there exists a disability at the level of my mind. Next, if the cycle is intact so far but I am unable to reach for the apple—if my mind is unable to command my body to perform the right action, or my body's response to my mind's command is inappropriate, as in some motor disorders—that too is obviously a disability.

All our actions are the consequence of such a cycle. Of course, the presence of the sense object may not be necessary for the mind to decide on a particular action. Simply the memory of the object is sufficient. To extend this to our example, I may not need to see the apple to want to eat it. Simply the memory of the apple can be enough to make me go to the kitchen, choose an apple, and eat it.

The source of disease is manifold. Many diseases arise partly from genetic and environmental causes, which are not under our complete control. For instance, a disease like bronchial asthma is affected by our genetic predisposition and by environmental factors. The acquisition of diabetes is, to an extent,

genetically determined. Hypertension can also result from a genetic predisposition and a stressful environment.

Whatever the cause of the disease, however, health maintenance involves preventing future diseases and alleviating existing ones. Both of these are implied in our translation of *cikitsa*: therapy to act against diseases, both existing ones and those that may occur in the future. Therapy is an active process. It is undeniable that our actions are the most important factor in both prevention and removal of disease.

Ayurveda and yoga state that the cause of disease or the means for therapy are threefold:

- The perception of sense objects by the mind (*artha*)
- The actions that we perform, based on our current perceptions or our memory of past experiences (karma)
- The changes that time brings, in us as individuals and in the environment around us (kala)

We have discussed the first two points in detail already. These two factors encompass our entire existence as individuals—our sensory perceptions, thoughts in the mind, and the actions that result from them. Changes in the connections we establish with the sense objects around us and the actions we do form the basis of any lifestyle change. Thus they are the key to effecting positive changes in our lives or adopting any form of therapy.

The third factor, kala, is where the genetic and environmental causes of disease or health fit in. The environment around us is in a state of constant change. Our body too is constantly changing at the cellular level—our genetic constitution plays an important role in determining the nature of such changes. Such changes are not a result of our activities. They will happen in some form whether we like them or not. They are the inevitable consequence of the passage of time.

When the cycle of perception and action proceeds without our active awareness, there is much room for abuse of the body and the mind. The pull of the senses is something we are all aware of. Since the mind is incessantly attracted to or repelled by the objects displayed to it by the senses, it continues to propel us into actions that could result in ill health.

However, when we pursue a course of action with awareness, it is possible to direct our senses and our body toward maintaining and restoring health.

CONNECTING YOGA AND AYURVEDA

A proper understanding of the connections between yoga and Ayurveda is essential for effective treatment of illnesses.

Asanas and the Treatment of Structural Imbalances

In structural problems like imbalances in strength, flexibility, skeletal alignment, or neuromuscular coordination, or other mechanical problems of the musculoskeletal system, movements (asanas) are most important in restoring health. This follows naturally from the nature of the problem. Breathing serves to support the movements we make. That is, the deciding factor is the type of movements to be made, on the basis of which we include the appropriate components of the breathing cycle, to enhance the effect of the movements or decrease any unwanted effects of some of the movements we use.

Diet, Breathing, and the Mind

Imbalances in the functioning of other body systems require that we first consider the person's diet and see if there exists a contributing or causative factor that we can remove or at least minimize. Because food, as we have discussed, has a direct influence on our body's qualities and functions and to some extent on the mind as well, it simply cannot be ignored.

Though both movements and breathing are integral to the practice of asanas, breathing is of greater importance than movement in addressing many disorders of body function such as hypertension or diabetes, or psychological disorders such as depression and anxiety. Therefore, we need to choose a body position in which the person is able to breathe freely, emphasizing the appropriate component of the breathing cycle. As was explained in the section on personalizing asana practice, this may translate to *pascimatanasana* in the case of a fit young woman; for an elderly man, it might mean bending forward while seated on a chair. In both cases, the emphasis should be on extended and complete exhalation. The movements and body positions are chosen to make such breathing possible and maximally effective in light of the person's capabilities or limitations.

That the mind affects various aspects of body function is well known and needs no elaboration. The most direct way to address problems in the mind is, of course, by changing the thought process itself. Breathing is a potent tool to influence the mind (in pranayama and asana). Bodily movements can be of help too, but they are secondary to breathing.

Diet, Breathing, and the Doshas

Ayurveda explains in detail how food affects the three doshas and various other body qualities and functions.

Classical yoga texts explain the connection between the various types of pranayama and the three doshas. Specific types of pranayama can be of use in decreasing the qualities of particular doshas when they are out of balance in the body. Also, these texts relate breathing to the qualities of heat and cold in the body. They classify the types of pranayama as heating and cooling and also suggest that inhalation through the right nostril is heating, while inhalation through the left nostril is cooling.

These specific connections between diet, breathing, and body qualities and functions is

one important reason they are of greater importance than body positions and movements in addressing functional problems in the body.

Asanas and Disease in Classical Yoga Texts

Classical texts on yoga such as the *Hatha-Yoga-Pradipika* describe several asanas and enumerate their benefits on the basis of Ayurveda—using the concept of the doshas, the same terminology for diseases, and the same list of body qualities and functions. However, they restrict themselves to stating that an asana can help restore balance among all three doshas or listing some diseases that are explained in Ayurveda. The important question here is, does the form of the asana alone confer the therapeutic benefits, or is it the breathing that is more important? The asana/disease correlation is usually based on simple anatomical grounds: Disorders of organ systems localized in the areas worked upon by the asana are sometimes listed as being cured by the asana. While this may be true to some extent, simple physical stimulation of body areas is not the focus of asana as a therapy, and it does not explain the considerable role that asanas play in addressing many disorders. Further, it is questionable whether a person suffering from these diseases will be able to do these asanas by rigidly adhering to their classic form. Even more doubtful is whether a sick person will benefit from such strenuous practices. It is important to note that commentaries on these texts generally clarify that these asanas are to be learned under the guidance of a teacher. Besides, these recommendations are mostly worded in a manner designed to inspire practitioners of yoga to practice with greater effort—they are not directed at an ill person. Much of their value is preventive. Finally, the texts that list these connections are in a poetic form and often highly exaggerated. You will find that they claim that several asanas will "cure all diseases." This is the style of composition, and the content must not be taken literally.

Ayurveda itself does not go into the details of asanas but merely recommends exercise as a component of several treatment regimens.

Agni: Connecting Asanas, Pranayama, and Diet

The importance of the agni is acknowledged in both yoga and Ayurveda. The primary purpose of all treatment, and an important goal of the practice of asanas, is to keep the agni functioning well. Here again, breathing is directly related to agni rather than specific types of movement. Inhalation helps to increase agni and activates metabolism, rather like fanning the flames of a fire. Exhalation, being a natural process of elimination, helps eliminate the toxins and wastes that dull the agni, and thus enables the agni to function better. In many functional disorders, it is important to ensure that exhalation is proper, even if inhalation is the component of breathing to be emphasized.

BRMHANA AND LANGHANA

Ayurveda mentions that all forms of therapy can be classified under two broad headings: those that nourish the body and add to the body tissues (*brmhana*) and those that remove from the body (*langhana*).

Most methods of therapy suggested in Ayurveda fall under langhana, including both palliative and eliminative methods, because, in both, we are mostly reducing some body quality that is out of balance. Brmhana includes only the measures like nourishing food and rejuvenating herbs, cool climate, pleasant surroundings, and so on, which, as we all know, can help to increase body mass. One reason for this is that most treatment in Ayurveda is viewed as a reduction or removal of imbalance, balance being a natural consequence of this process. Another reason is that treatment is basically dependent on the status of the agni. Langhana helps to increase the function of agni by removing the wastes (*ama*) that impair the functioning of the agni. For brmhana to be effective, the agni has to be functioning properly. Otherwise, even if we consume nourishing foodstuffs and herbs, they will not be of use to our body, because, as we have discussed, agni is what allows food to become transformed into body tissues. In many disease states, langhana is usually required first to remove the blockage in the functioning of the agni. Only then will brmhana be possible at all. That is why Ayurvedic texts suggest that even in a situation where brmhana is necessary, it may be good to start with mild langhana first. However, the opposite does not apply: Brmhana is not to be done for a person who requires langhana.

In yoga, the application of brmhana and langhana is an extension of the concepts outlined in Ayurveda.

There exist pairs of opposites in the body, breathing, mind, and food. Some major pairs are forward- and backward-bending movements (body), inhalation and exhalation (breath), activity and relaxation (mind), and heating and cooling (food). Classifying all such opposites under brmhana and langhana—that is, extending the classification of brmhana and langhana to encompass a wide variety of opposites in body, breathing, mind, and food—greatly increases the potential for confusion and also further dilutes the specificity of the approach. This is because it amounts to grouping qualities in body, breathing, mind, and food together when this is not always recommended in therapy.

For example, consider an overweight middle-aged person with high blood pressure. If he or she can do it, we would suggest an active asana practice with emphasis on extended exhalation. Should such a sequence be called a brmhana practice, because of the activating effect of vigorous movement, or should it be classified as a langhana practice because of the emphasis on extended exhalation?

It is difficult to propose an approach to high blood pressure based on this classification. For a lean elderly person with high blood pressure, the suggested asana practice would

emphasize simple, relaxing forward-bending movements and extended exhalation—which would translate into a langhana approach. The most consistent point in the approach to hypertension in any individual is the emphasis on exhalation. Hypertension is a disorder of Vata and is aggravated by increased mental activity. Therefore, exhalation and not inhalation is the component of the breathing cycle to be emphasized. This example shows why breathing is often more important and more directly involved in the therapy of functional disorders. The movements we do in asanas will vary depending on individual factors.

In the case of depression, the approach is to activate the person's mind. The emphasis is commonly on inhalation and backward-bending movements, but we could achieve this activation in several other ways depending on the individual. For example, we could suggest that the ratio of inhalation and exhalation be made equal, or we could suspend breathing after exhalation to provoke the succeeding inhalation. Also, although in depression the primary aim is to reduce the tamas in the person's mind, we do not want to end up also increasing rajas. Therefore, we might end the practice with deep, extended exhalation. If you see this in an asana practice, do not make the mistake of thinking that it is brmhana (backward-bending movements) for the body and brmhana/langhana (inhalation/exhalation) for the mind.

There is no brmhana or langhana for the mind in Ayurveda. The classification applies only to the body. A classification based on activity and relaxation is almost invariably misleading, because it is oversimplified. To deal with the mind, the appropriate classification of mental states, thoughts, and emotions is only that of the three gunas—sattva, rajas, and tamas. To continue our example of depression, the lack of activity in the mind could be due to a feeling of despair and hopelessness; in some cases, the lack of activity could be due to anger and frustration. We must look at the circumstances and the person's mind before suggesting any approach. A very clear understanding of how the thinking process operates, how emotions are connected to each other, and so on, is essential in dealing with psychological illness.

When we relate food to the other constituents of body, breath, and mind under this classification, there is the possibility of further confusion. The classification of brmhana and langhana as proposed in Ayurveda makes sense because Ayurveda deals mainly with the effects of food and medicine on the body. Since food is the only way to directly add to the body, it is actually the only way to bring about brmhana—to nourish the body and increase its mass. If you do not eat well, you will not experience a brmhana effect no matter what your yoga practice may be. That is why Ayurveda groups all exercise under langhana—as we all know, exercise (of the aerobic kind) helps to reduce body weight by burning energy. Therefore, from an Ayurvedic point of view, all asana practice is langhana. However, exercise or asana practice results in better functioning

of agni. Brmhana is the result of eating the right food when the agni is functioning well. This is why Ayurveda also suggests that some langhana may be a good idea before brmhana.

For example, consider the case of a thin person with fairly severe asthma. In asthma, the airways are narrowed, resulting in obstruction of the outflow of air and retention of air in the lungs. Therefore, the suggested asana and pranayama practice should generally emphasize exhalation. In the diet, heavy, Kapha-related foods should be decreased and substituted with lighter foodstuffs. As a consequence of these changes, the functioning of the agni will usually improve, and the person may put on a few pounds to reach a more ideal weight. Note that here we are suggesting an emphasis on exhalation (langhana), with lighter foodstuffs (langhana), but the net result is an increase in body mass (brmhana). From the Ayurvedic viewpoint, there is no contradiction here. Lighter food can help to reduce the production of wastes and toxins that impair the functioning of the agni. This improved functioning of the agni later results in brmhana because the person's food is better utilized. When we extend this concept to body, breathing, and mind, however, we have overlapping and confusing results.

Whatever classification we adopt, a clear understanding of the relationship between body and mind and their relationships with breathing and food is essential in order to apply yoga and Ayurveda effectively in the treatment of any illness.

YOGA THERAPY IN CLASSICAL YOGA TEXTS

Classical yoga texts describe diseases using terminology borrowed from Ayurveda. Ayurveda uses only the model of the three doshas everywhere to present an approach to physical health. Both yoga and Ayurveda use the three gunas to present an approach to mental health. We have outlined both these models in chapter 1.

One important reason for the confusion surrounding many classical yoga texts, except for the *Yoga-Sutras*, is their mixed content: They contain everything from tantric sex practices and cutting the frenulum of the tongue to guidelines on pranayama and standard descriptions borrowed from nondualistic philosophy. This is reflective of the varied sources and wide scope of the information in these texts. These yoga texts are to be read and interpreted cautiously, not taken literally.

You may come across two important concepts—*cakras* and *koshas*—in both classical texts and contemporary books on yoga. A detailed explanation of these concepts is beyond the scope of this book. However, as we explain briefly in the interview in appendix C, it is important to understand that these are not approaches to yoga therapy.

Case Studies for the Yoga Therapist

8

THE CASE studies presented here illustrate how the theory described in the previous chapters is applied in a therapeutic setting. It is not helpful merely to state the solution in a specific case without adequately explaining the approach. Asanas, as we have said, are especially important in the treatment of structural problems. Therefore, this chapter primarily presents examples of problems of body structure, along with a few cases of constipation and menstrual problems. Major illnesses like diabetes or hypertension are not addressed here. In the therapy of such disorders, many factors need to be considered, especially those related to diet, lifestyle, and the mind, any of which may be as important as the practice of asanas or pranayama in a particular case. A detailed consideration of these is beyond the scope of this book.

The first case illustrates how the various principles related to the practice of asanas—the characteristics of movement and breathing, observation, sequencing, and personalization—are applied in a therapeutic situation. The condition used as an example is inguinal hernia.

In designing an asana program for treating a specific condition, we first need to know two things: the movements likely to be useful in addressing that condition and the components of the breathing cycle that will be useful in addressing that condition. Keeping this knowledge in mind, we assess the characteristics of the person and the severity of the condition and then design the asana program using the principles of sequencing and personalization.

In therapy, problem-specific guidelines play a major role in deciding our strategy. An

> **Asana as therapy—important steps in the decision-making process:**
> - Know what movements and breathing will be useful for that condition.
> - Know the progression to be incorporated in movement and breathing.
> - Observe and assess the characteristics of the person.
> - Assess the intensity of the problem.
> - Decide the starting point, the broad outline of the sequence, and the required personalization.
> - Continue to observe and assess as the person practices, and further optimize.

idea of the nature of movements, breathing, and diet and lifestyle changes that will be useful for a particular problem can usually be arrived at through analysis. Even more important is to know what will aggravate or worsen the condition. We must try to eliminate or at least avoid these factors.

INGUINAL HERNIA

Hernia is a protrusion of the contents of a cavity through its walls due to a weakness or defect in the wall. Inguinal hernia, a common complaint seen in surgical practice, involves protrusion of some abdominal contents—such as a loop of the intestine—through the inguinal canal, situated slightly above and lateral to the pubic bone. Inguinal hernia is more common in males, and when it occurs in adulthood it is often associated with lax abdominal muscles.

Asana practice is very useful in preventing and treating inguinal hernia. It also can complement surgery effectively, especially postop-

eratively, to avoid recurrence and to make sure that hernia does not develop on the other side. The discussion below applies to cases of uncomplicated, reducible inguinal hernia.

Problem-Specific Guidelines: The Dos

In a case of inguinal hernia, building abdominal muscle strength is the most important goal of asana practice. To increase the strength of the abdominal muscles, we must make them contract. But this creates a problem: Contracting the abdominal muscles increases the intraabdominal pressure, which can cause herniation.

We need to select the movements that will be most useful and also know which ones to avoid. We also need to decide which component of the breathing cycle to emphasize. In short, we need to analyze the following characteristics of the movement and breathing and select the most favorable options:

- The direction of movement (forward, backward, twisting, or lateral) to use

- The body position (standing, seated, lying, or inverted) from which the movements are made
- The component of the breathing cycle (inhalation, exhalation, suspension, or retention) to emphasize

Direction of movement. Backward-bending movements stretch the front of the body and therefore stretch rather than contract the abdominal muscles. Twisting and lateral-bending movements also partially stretch the abdominal muscles. Gentle twisting movements are useful when done after exhalation, but only in the later stages of the practice. Only forward-bending movements can help achieve sustained and effective contraction of the abdominal muscles. Therefore, in cases of inguinal hernia, the asana practice should emphasize forward-bending movements, with graded increase in the contraction of the abdominal muscles (fig. 8.1).

Body position. When the abdominal muscles contract, the contents of the abdomen are compressed and the intraabdominal pressure increases. This increase in pressure can aggravate the hernia. Therefore, when designing a

Favorable   **Unfavorable**

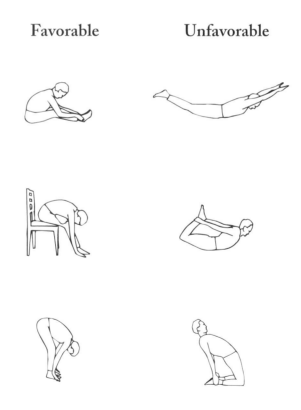

Fig. 8.1. Some examples of favorable and unfavorable asanas for inguinal hernia based on the direction of movement.

practice to make the abdominal muscles contract, we must choose body positions and breathing that will minimize the corresponding increase in intraabdominal pressure. In positions where the trunk is upright (standing and seated positions), gravity pulls the abdominal contents downward, and the pressure in the lower abdomen is greater. In the lying position, however, the abdominal contents are moved away from the anterior abdominal wall by gravity, and this reduces their tendency to bulge out at the front of the body. Further, in forward bending from standing and seated positions, the weight of the trunk compresses the abdomen, in addition to the compressive force exerted by the contracting abdominal muscles. Therefore, the compressive force on the abdominal contents is greater when forward-bending movements are done from standing and seated positions than when they are done from the lying position. Since other muscles groups in the body are relaxed in the lying position, this allows the person to judge more accurately the degree to which the abdominal muscles are contracting, thus making graded contraction of the abdominal muscles easier to achieve.

However, when the person is lying on the back, the legs must not be extended, as this will stretch the abdominal muscles. Bending the legs at the knees will relax the abdominal muscles, allow free breathing, and permit controlled, graded contraction of those muscles. Therefore, in the initial stages, the ideal position to start working with inguinal hernia is the semisupine position: lying on the back with the knees bent.

Forward-bending movements from the seated and standing positions are useful when done with appropriate breathing, but they are more strenuous than forward-bending movements done from the lying position. Therefore, they should be introduced gradually as the person progresses. The condition of the person and the severity of the problem largely determine to what extent seated and standing forward bends can be used in the practice. In a relatively young and active person, forward-bending movements like *uttanasana* to a chair or even complete *uttanasana* can be introduced early on.

Inversions are ideal for inguinal hernia. In inverted positions, the weight of the abdominal contents is completely shifted away from the inguinal (lower abdominal) region. In this position, the abdominal muscles can be strongly contracted with minimal risk of causing herniation. There are two classic inverted positions used in asanas: shoulder stand and headstand. Shoulder stand is the position of choice in inguinal hernia. In headstand, the legs lean backward slightly at the hips. This helps in maintaining the position with less effort, using the passive tension of ligaments instead of active muscle contraction to hold the body in place. This backward tilt of the legs stretches the abdomen, making headstand similar in some respects to a backward-bending movement. In shoulder stand, however, the legs are not tilted backward. Instead, it is easier to bend them forward. This makes shoulder stand similar to a forward-bending movement, but with the advantages of inversion.

Breathing. Correct breathing is the key to the success of asana practice in working with inguinal hernia. Exhalation is the component of the breathing cycle to be emphasized. Exhalation and suspension after exhalation help to contract the abdominal muscles. They also naturally complement forward-bending movements. In all cases of inguinal hernia, extended exhalation and suspension after exhalation with conscious contraction of the abdominal muscles is the starting point. The person must be taught to breathe like this in the semisupine position, before it is introduced in other movements. It is vital to ensure that people are able to do complete and extended exhalation before proceeding to teach other movements. If not, they may hold their breath or exhale incompletely in forward-bending movements. This will lead to an increase in intraabdominal pressure and will aggravate the condition or at least result in a lack of progress. Figure 8.2 summarizes the movements and breathing that are favorable and unfavorable in inguinal hernia.

Breathing also plays an important role in minimizing the unfavorable effect of some of the movements we include in the asana practice. We use asanas like *dvipadapitham* to prepare the person to do shoulder stand. In shoulder stand, the neck is completely flexed—bent forward so that the chin is in contact with, or very close to, the front of the chest. Also, the weight of the trunk is borne partially by the arms and elbows, but some of it is transferred to the shoulders, neck, and upper back. Shoulder stand places

Favorable

BREATHING	MOVEMENT
• Extended exhalation	• Forward bends
• Suspension after exhalation	• Gentle twists (later)
• Use of bandhas	
• Use of sound	

Unfavorable

BREATHING	MOVEMENT
• Inhalation	• Strong backward bends
• Holding after inhalation	• Deep twists
• Rapid breathing	• Lateral bends
• Kapalabhati pranayama	

Fig. 8.2. Movements and breathing favorable or unfavorable to the treatment of inguinal hernia.

considerable stress on the neck, bending it forward by force, and therefore it requires careful preparation of the neck, shoulders, and upper back. Moreover, breathing in this position is not easy. The bent position of the neck hinders free breathing.

Now observe the position of the neck in *dvipadapitham*. It is flexed as in shoulder stand; however, in *dvipadapitham*, the stress on the neck is less because the neck is flexed less and also because the weight of the trunk does not rest on it—the position is maintained by contraction of the back and thigh muscles. Thus *dvipadapitham* is similar to shoulder stand but much less strenuous. It can therefore serve as a preparation for shoulder stand, preparing the neck, shoulders, and upper back and familiarizing the person with breathing when the neck is flexed.

In a case of inguinal hernia, however, *dvipadapitham* is an undesirable position. It stretches the abdominal muscles rather than contracting them. It is a backward-bending movement, which is not useful in dealing with inguinal hernia. Yet *dvipadapitham* is very important as a preparation for shoulder stand, which is of considerable benefit in inguinal hernia. Therefore, we face the question of how to maximize the useful component of *dvipadapitham*—the work on the upper back, shoulders, and neck—while minimizing the unfavorable stretching of the abdominal muscles.

We can do this by skillfully modifying the breathing. *Dvipadapitham* is a movement that opens out the chest and stretches the front of the body, and it is usually done on inhalation. Inhalation enhances the effect of *dvipadapitham* in stretching the muscle groups in the front of the body. But in inguinal hernia, we do not want to emphasize this effect. Instead, we want to avoid the synergism of inhalation with the back-bending movement in stretching the abdominal muscles. Therefore, we restrict the length of inhalation and instead stress exhalation. We can even reverse the normal combination of breathing and movement—we can teach the person to make the backward-bending movement into *dvipadapitham* on exhalation. Then, we instruct the person to stay in that position, take in a short inhalation, and do extended exhalation. Further, we also ensure that the person restricts the inhalation to the chest as much as possible and consciously prevents the abdomen from coming outward on inhalation. The short duration of inhalation helps in this. Figure 8.3 provides a summary of the role *dvipadapitham* can play in treating inguinal hernia.

This is a classic example of how a skillful use of breathing can enhance certain effects of a movement and minimize others.

In summary, when dealing with inguinal hernia, we start with emphasizing exhalation done in the supine position with legs bent. We gradually introduce some standing and seated positions as the person becomes stronger, to maintain balance in the practice. We should prepare the person to reach the stage where he or she can do *uddiyana-bandha* in shoulder stand. This process may take weeks or even

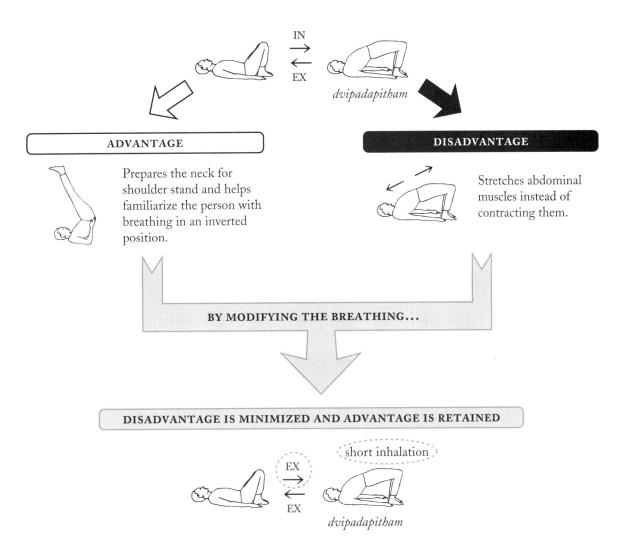

Fig. 8.3. Using breathing to enhance the positive effects and minimize the unwanted effects of movement: the role of *dvipadapitham* in treating inguinal hernia.

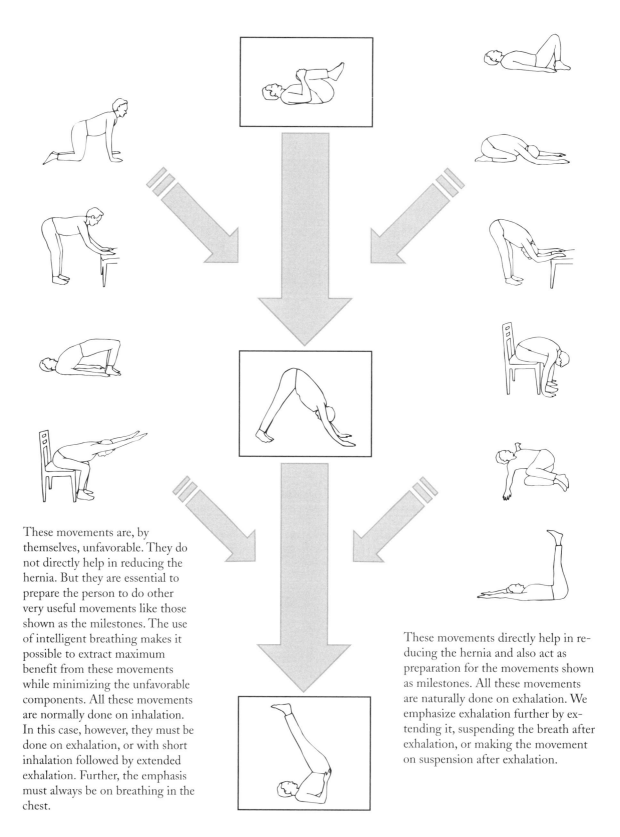

These movements are, by themselves, unfavorable. They do not directly help in reducing the hernia. But they are essential to prepare the person to do other very useful movements like those shown as the milestones. The use of intelligent breathing makes it possible to extract maximum benefit from these movements while minimizing the unfavorable components. All these movements are normally done on inhalation. In this case, however, they must be done on exhalation, or with short inhalation followed by extended exhalation. Further, the emphasis must always be on breathing in the chest.

These movements directly help in reducing the hernia and also act as preparation for the movements shown as milestones. All these movements are naturally done on exhalation. We emphasize exhalation further by extending it, suspending the breath after exhalation, or making the movement on suspension after exhalation.

Fig. 8.4. Progression in movement in the therapy of inguinal hernia. The asanas in the boxes in the central column can be considered milestones toward which the other asanas lead.

months, depending upon the person's capacity, condition, and commitment to the practice. Figure 8.4 summarizes the progression in movement to be employed in dealing with inguinal hernia. Figure 8.5 outlines the progression to be followed in breathing.

Sound. Sound can be used effectively in contracting the abdominal muscles. Asking the

person to recite a sound aloud after exhalation will intensify the contraction of the abdominal muscles.

Problem-Specific Guidelines: The Don'ts

Strong backward-bending movements like *salabhasana* must be completely avoided. But, as the person progresses, gentle backward-

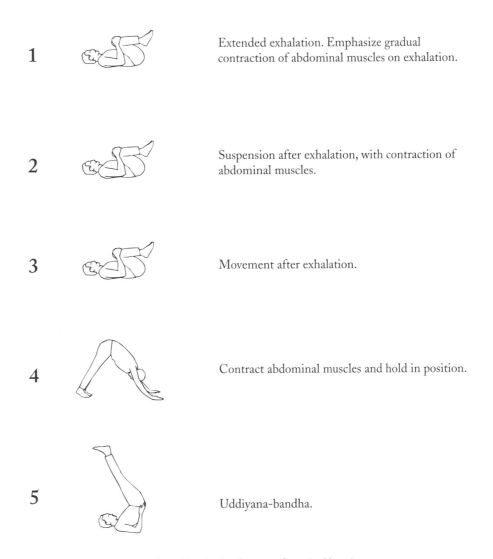

1 — Extended exhalation. Emphasize gradual contraction of abdominal muscles on exhalation.

2 — Suspension after exhalation, with contraction of abdominal muscles.

3 — Movement after exhalation.

4 — Contract abdominal muscles and hold in position.

5 — Uddiyana-bandha.

Fig. 8.5. Progression in breathing in the therapy of inguinal hernia.

bending movements are necessary to avoid an unbalanced practice. As we pass from the stage of healing to the stage of strengthening, backward bends of increasing intensity can gradually be introduced.

Forward-bending movements done on inhalation or while holding the breath—without letting the breath out—are also to be avoided absolutely. These will increase the intra-abdominal pressure and worsen the condition. Emphasizing inhalation is itself unwise.

Strenuous forms of pranayama like kapalabhati, in which the abdomen is moved in and out rapidly, must be avoided.

The Role of Ayurveda

It is important to prevent the development of constipation in a person with inguinal hernia. That is, the function of apana vata must be maintained without disturbance. Staying in one location and avoiding excessive traveling are helpful. Constipation is discussed further below.

ACHES AND PAINS

The cases presented in this section can be divided into two broad groups on the basis of important differences in our therapeutic approach. The first group includes cases of aches and pains in otherwise healthy people primarily from structural causes—imbalances in strength, flexibility, and alignment—commonly brought about by excessive use, disuse, or abuse of a particular body area. The emphasis in the therapeutic approach is on correcting the particular imbalance through the practice of a carefully designed asana program. Mostly, Ayurveda plays a supportive role in addressing these problems, for, although changes in diet and lifestyle form an important part of any yoga and Ayurveda therapy, the structural nature of the problem dictates an emphasis on asanas.

The second group of cases are those in which the aches and pains are associated with or caused by an underlying pathological process—a degenerative or autoimmune condition like osteoarthritis or rheumatoid arthritis, for example. In these cases, there is a significant role for Ayurveda; diet changes and some herbs can be very useful. The approach we use in designing a yoga program for these conditions is also somewhat different, as we are attempting to resolve not a simple imbalance in structure in a particular body area but a more pervasive functional disorder.

In dealing with any ache or pain, some general points must always be considered. First, we need to know whether movement increases or decreases the pain. That is, the relation of movements to the severity and occurrence of the pain must be clear. Next, it is wise to always inquire if the person is taking painkillers. Pain is an indicator of tissue damage, a signal that must be respected. Painkillers can make it difficult for people to recognize if exercise is increasing their pain. Sometimes exercise can be detrimental and only rest will help the body heal. In such cases, we may have to restrict ourselves to simple breathing exercises and mental techniques. It is also useful to consider the relation of the pain to other factors, such as food intake, time of day, digestion, or the presence of occasional swelling.

In asana practice for aches and pains, it is advisable to steer clear of movements or body positions that place stress on the affected body part, especially in the early stages. Such movements can be introduced gradually, as the person progresses and the pain diminishes. In the case of knee pain, for example, it is important to avoid movements or body positions that apply pressure or stress on the knees, such as a cross-legged sitting posture or asanas such as *matsyasana*, *paryankasana*, *padmasana*, and *dhanurasana*. If there is hip pain, staying in asanas like *ardha uttanasana*, *virabhadrasana*, and *ardha salabhasana* can aggravate it. So can asanas done with straight legs. In the case of shoulder pain, asanas like *adhomukhasvanasana*, *urdhvamukhasvanasana*, *dhanurasana*, headstand, shoulder stand, and *ardha matsyendrasana* are to be used judiciously. Staying in positions in which the arms are raised overhead also stresses the shoulders. Such guidelines can all be derived by an analysis of the body position, and their suitability for the person can be judged using the principles outlined in the earlier section on asanas.

Dynamic movements can be useful in relieving the stress caused by static positions. Therefore, when there is stiffness of joints or a particular body area as a result of remaining in the same position for extended periods, the asana practice can include movements that alternately but gently bend and stretch that body area.

The knees, back, and neck are three common sites of pain. Ironically, many practitioners of yoga in the West suffer from back, neck, and knee pain. The Western lifestyle has many contributing factors: playing sports, frequent travel in automobiles, and the sedentary nature of many people's work, for example. Classical yoga asanas were proposed in the context of the radically different lifestyle found in rural India centuries ago. Even today in rural India, it is common for people to sit on the floor in a cross-legged position or squat on the floor for several hours a day. Such people can assume asanas like the lotus pose relatively easily. Inserting the same asanas into the exercise schedule of Westerners without adequate preparation can aggravate or even cause structural problems.

The occurrence of uncomplicated aches and pains is common, especially with increasing age; often it is due to lack of regular use, sometimes to improper use. In these situations, the person is healthy and there is no significant structural or functional abnormality underlying the problem. Usually, in such cases, the principles pertaining to observation, sequencing, and personalization are sufficient to design an effective asana program.

We have emphasized the need to start from where the person is. In the sections on observation, sequencing, and personalization, we spoke of the starting point in terms of characteristics such as strength and flexibility. In therapeutic situations such as those involving back pain, the starting point often depends not on such personal factors but on the severity of the specific problem. On this basis, we

General guidelines for dealing with aches and pains:
- Look into the history of the problem and try to ascertain the cause of the pain.
- Inquire and also test whether movement increases or decreases the pain.
- Check whether the person is on painkillers.
- Start from where the person is.
- Steer clear of stressful body positions.

can place all cases into three broad groups. In the first group are people in fairly severe pain or in bed, maybe after corrective surgery. That is, the pain is a major hindrance that makes it difficult or impossible for them to perform normal activities. In the second group are people who are able to carry out their normal activities but suffer from chronic pain—that is, the pain occurs predictably, every day, although it may vary in severity. The third group consists of people in whom the pain occurs intermittently, perhaps caused by greater than normal activity. Their condition may worsen if proper preventive action is not taken.

Back Pain

Back pain is certainly the most important of all the aches and pains discussed in this sec-

tion. Indeed, there are few adults who have not experienced some form of back pain at some time in their lives.

An asana program for back pain has three important goals:

- Strengthening the abdominal muscles
- Stretching the hamstrings
- Strengthening the back muscles

Ancient yoga texts suggest asanas like *navasana* to strengthen the abdominal muscles, *pascimatanasana* to stretch the hamstrings, and *salabhasana* to strengthen the back muscles. These are strenuous asanas. Many fit people cannot do them as they are depicted in the yoga texts, let alone a person suffering from back pain. Such asanas are suggested with prevention in mind, not as

Three grades of aches and pains relevant to the designing of an asana practice:
- Severe pain. Unable to carry on normal daily activities.
- Chronic pain that occurs predictably but may vary in intensity. Able to do normal activities.
- Intermittent pain precipitated by greater than normal activity.

therapeutic measures. They are the goal, and the asana program must aim to gradually lead the person toward these asanas. Old age, decreased fitness, and severe back pain can all limit the progress we make, and attaining the ideal may never be possible for a particular person. That does not matter. What is important is progress toward the ideal. For example, doing *navasana* may require a degree of abdominal muscle strength and general fitness that a person may never reach, but the same person can definitely increase his or her abdominal strength through similar but simpler movements and breathing. Again, it is vital to keep in mind that the goal is relative to the starting point. To determine the starting point and the further steps required, we must consider several factors:

1. General characteristics of the person
   a. Age
   b. Height: short, average, or tall
   c. Weight: lean, normal, or overweight
   d. Occupation: standing or seated
2. History of the problem. Try to gain an idea of the causes of the problem in the person's lifestyle. Many cases will fall under more than one of the categories below, but this information is nevertheless important.
   a. Injury (e.g., from sports)
   b. Chronic overuse (e.g., dancers, gymnasts, and others placing constant repetitive stress on their back and hips)
   c. Chronic disuse (e.g., resulting from aging or sickness)
3. Relationship of the occurrence and severity

of back pain to the following:
   a. Body position (Is the pain aggravated or relieved by standing, seated, or lying positions? More simply, which body position is most comfortable?)
   b. Time of day (Is the pain better or worse in the morning or evening?)
   c. Activity (Does the pain increase or decrease with activity?)
   d. Rest (Does rest relieve the pain? In other words, is the pain better or worse on awaking in the morning? Is it difficult to get out of bed because of the pain or stiffness?)
   e. Food (Does eating affect the nature or severity of the pain?)
4. Other physical conditions
   a. Is the pain worse in flexion or extension?
   b. How strong is the person?
   c. How flexible is the person?
   d. Are there structural misalignments present (e.g., asymmetry)?
   e. Is the person likely to tolerate pain well?
5. Severity of the back pain
   a. Is the person in bed because of severe pain or recent surgery?
   b. Is the person suffering from chronic pain but able to carry out normal activities?
   c. Is the pain intermittent and brought on by strenuous activities?
6. Other associated factors, including pregnancy, heart problems, asthma, hypertension, scoliosis, kyphosis or lordosis, neck pain, shoulder pain, hip pain, current medications, and so on.

Case Study 1: Knee Pain

John, an American, age thirty-five, was an architect. Tall and lean, he had been interested in yoga for several years and had read many books on the subject and attended some classes. He was practicing asanas for one hour every morning and complained that he often developed pain in both knees at the end of his practice. The pain was not associated with swelling or any other symptoms.

I observed his movements in a few simple asanas and found that his low back and hamstrings were stiff, but his back was strong and there was no asymmetry in his spine. I then elicited the details of his current practice. He said that he was doing several asanas shown in figure 8.6 regularly, staying in each for a few minutes.

Even with adequate preparation, a practice that included all these asanas would place considerable stress on his knees, and he was doing them all without adequate preparation. The stress he was placing on his knees was further compounded by the stiffness in his back and legs. He was forcing himself into these positions and staying in them trying to use his strength to overcome his lack of flexibility.

I suggested that he avoid such asanas and work with movements that would increase the flexibility of his back. To do this, I advised that he use forward bends with proper breathing to stretch his low back muscles. I told him that as he continued to practice regularly, the new sequence of movements would gradually increase his flexibility. They would

also place less strain on his knees so he would not have any knee pain after his practice. In time, he could add more backward-bending movements to his practice to maintain the strength of his back. The asanas I suggested to help increase the flexibility of his back and hamstrings are shown in figure 8.7.

Case Study 1: Knee pain
Key observations and assessment
- Fit young man with strong back and stiff hamstrings.
- Current asana practice includes asanas that strain the knees.

Principal suggestions
- Stop current practice.
- Use only asanas that do not place stress on the knees.
- Use forward-bending asanas with long exhalation to stretch the lower back.

Case Study 2: Knee Pain

Sheela was a talented exponent of classical Indian dance, with many performances to her credit. She was thirty-four years old, five feet, five inches tall, and weighed 115 pounds. Lately she had developed knee pain and was deeply concerned by it, as it would affect her career. She planned to perform at a dance festival in a few months and was worried that her knee pain would prevent her from doing so.

She told me that she practiced dancing for two hours, asanas for thirty minutes, and meditation for fifteen minutes every day. Her asana practice consisted mainly of standing forward bends, *paryankasana*, and *matsyasana*. She did meditation seated in *padmasana*. Observing her in some simple movements

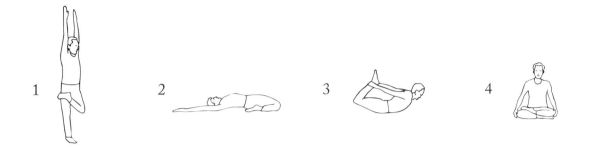

Fig. 8.6. Case Study 1: Asanas that were placing stress on the knees.

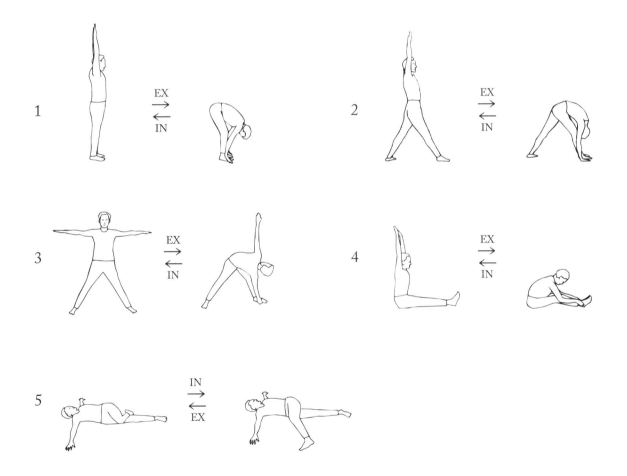

Fig. 8.7. Case Study 1: Suggested asanas to reduce stress on the knees and increase back flexibility.

and positions, I noticed that the arches of her feet had fallen. She was also very flexible, especially in her hips, and her back was weak. She had a long, slender neck, and her neck muscles seemed to lack adequate strength.

The form of dance she practiced involved stamping her feet on the ground, heavily and repeatedly. This motion also places considerable stress on the knees, predisposing the dancer to knee pain. Sheela suffered from knee and foot pain. Her dancing was causing her to use her feet and knees excessively, subjecting them to a greater degree of force than advisable. She was exacerbating the problem by doing asanas like *matsyasana* and *padmasana*, under the misguided impression that they would help reduce her knee pain. The contribution of her profession to her problem could not be denied, but neither could it be avoided. Therefore, I had to design her asana practice to oppose the deleterious effect her dancing could be having on her body structure.

I designed her asana practice with four primary objectives in mind:

- Reducing the stress on her knees
- Opposing further deterioration in the arches of her feet
- Strengthening her back
- Avoiding increasing the flexibility of her hips any further

Consequently, I reduced the number of standing positions in her practice and used movements shown in figure 8.8.

Case Study 3: Hip Pain

Thomas, forty-five years old, was a writer, five feet, seven inches tall, and weighing 130 pounds. He had injured his right knee in an accident six months earlier and now felt stiffness in his hips, especially on the right side. The long hours of sitting at his desk also added to his problem. He was in the habit of doing some stretching exercises for thirty minutes in the morning, but he felt that they were not of much help.

Simply from observing the way he walked, using his left leg more than his right, I thought he might have some problem with the right side of his body. This was confirmed when he related the details of his problem. Though he had now recovered and no longer needed to rest, he had developed the habit of protecting his right leg from too much weight. Therefore, he was placing more of his weight on his left leg, leaning a little to that side as he walked.

Testing him in simple movements, I found that the left side of his back was very stiff, more so than the right side. The asana practice I designed for him included asymmetrical forward-bending movements from the standing position (variations of *parsva uttanasana*) and other asymmetrical movements to achieve maximum work on each side of his back (fig. 8.9). Apart from his asana practice in the morning, I suggested that he take a ten-minute break twice a day and practice the same asymmetrical forward bend he did in the morning.

He felt much better in a week and was

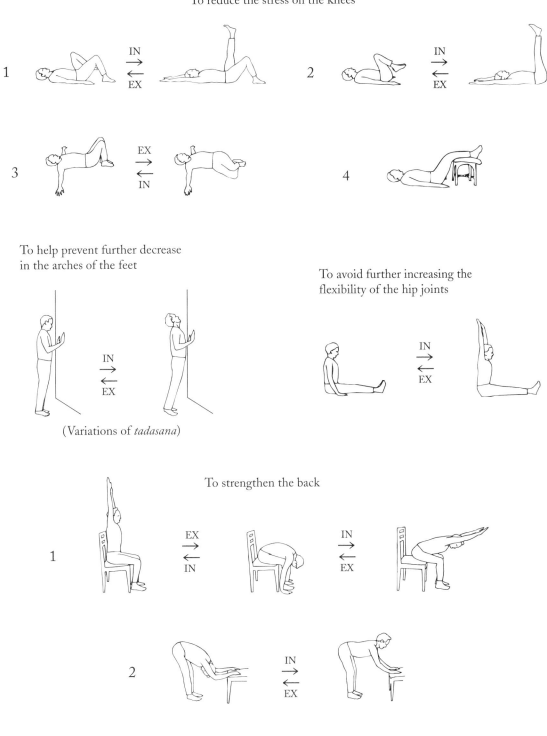

To reduce the stress on the knees

To help prevent further decrease
in the arches of the feet

(Variations of *tadasana*)

To avoid further increasing the
flexibility of the hip joints

To strengthen the back

Fig. 8.8. Case Study 2: Asanas used to address various needs.

almost normal in three months. His pattern of walking became more balanced, because he now felt confident about placing weight on his right leg.

> **Case Study 3: Hip pain/stiffness**
> *Key observations and assessment*
> - Tall, well-built, middle-aged man recovering from injury to right knee.
> - Places more weight on left leg when walking.
> - Lower back very stiff, left side more than right.
> - Sitting for long hours (occupational) has contributed to development of stiffness.
>
> *Principal suggestions*
> - Include asymmetrical forward- and backward-bending movements in asana practice.
> - Practice simple, asymmetrical standing forward-bending movements during short breaks from work.

Case Study 4: Shoulder Pain

Rekha, thirty-eight years old, five feet, five inches tall, and weighing 125 pounds, was a dentist. She had two children in school and was extremely busy with her work at home and at her clinic. She came to me with pain in her right shoulder. She had been putting up with the pain for three months and pushing herself to avoid falling behind in her work. I first suggested some simple movements to relax her shoulders, upper back, and neck. The entire practice was done from lying and seated positions, as she was on her feet throughout her working hours. I told her to apply oil on her right shoulder and massage it gently every day. I also taught her some simple movements to be done three times a day,

while taking a five-minute break during her working hours (fig. 8.10).

I also suggested some basic diet changes, mainly aimed at reducing the heavy, oily food she was having for breakfast and dinner.

The exercise and oil massage were of only marginal help. They decreased the pain, but only temporarily. Consequently, Rekha visited me again in a month, her shoulder pain practically undiminished. She also said that she was unable to stick to the diet changes I had suggested. I then gave her an Ayurvedic medicine to be taken orally. Combined with a stricter adherence to a healthier diet and more regularly timed meals, this had some effect. The pain decreased in severity, but she still suffered from occasional shooting pains.

It was clear that Rekha's work was aggravating her shoulder pain. On the rare occasions that she took a day off, her pain decreased by the evening. I told her that the only way to help her shoulder heal was to give it rest. After three more months and two more visits, she finally agreed to take three weeks off from her work. She was much better at the end of her holiday. Rest was the key factor in her case.

Case Study 5: Frozen Shoulder

Vanessa, forty-eight years old, was a physician at a leading hospital, with a busy private practice as well. She was tall and well built. The range of movement in her left shoulder had gradually decreased over a period of six months to the point where she found herself unable to lift her arm more than a few inches

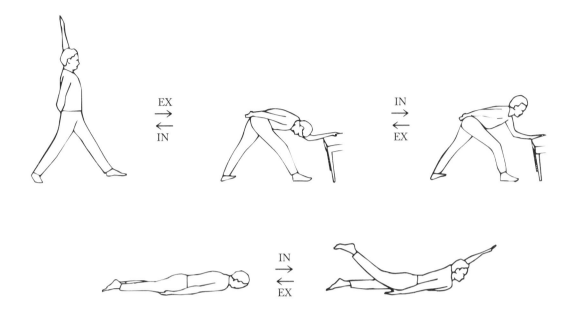

Fig. 8.9. Case Study 3: Standing and lying asymmetrical asanas for hip pain.

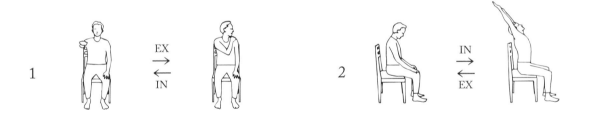

Fig. 8.10. Case Study 4: Simple movements for shoulder pain to be practiced three times a day during five-minute breaks.

above shoulder level. She was healthy in all other respects. At this point, she approached me to see if yoga could help what she described as a classic case of frozen shoulder. She was new to yoga but brought much sincerity to her practice.

In such cases, we have to restrict the range of arm movement to what the person is comfortable with. Later, as the condition improves, progressively greater ranges of movement can be introduced. In fact, it is usually possible to increase the range of movement to some extent within each session. The improvement, however, may not last for long after a single session; the benefit accrues over a period of time.

Vanessa found raising her left arm to the front much easier than raising it to the side. I suggested a practice that incorporated gradually increasing movement of her left arm. Her back was quite strong, but her upper back was stiff, so I included some simple arching movements to work on her upper back. Deep, extended breathing was a vital component of her practice; I told her that her attention should always be on her breath.

Ayurveda views this problem as arising from a blockage in movement, a character of Vata, caused by cold, attributed to Kapha. Therefore, I recommended that she apply an oil to her shoulder that according to Ayurveda would have a heating effect, and

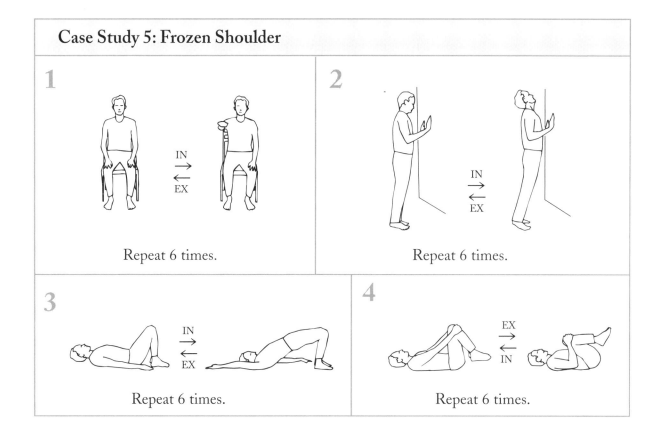

Case Study 5: Frozen Shoulder

1   IN → ← EX   Repeat 6 times.

2   IN → ← EX   Repeat 6 times.

3   IN → ← EX   Repeat 6 times.

4   EX → ← IN   Repeat 6 times.

massage it gently every day. Following this, she was to have a hot bath.

Vanessa was slightly surprised that the practice I gave her was so short and that my other suggestions were so simple. She told me that she had come to me with a very different idea about yoga. However, she practiced regularly and sincerely and was pleasantly surprised by the improvement in her shoulder.

Case Study 5: Guidelines for working with frozen shoulder
- Restrict the range of the movement to the limits the person finds comfortable.
- Include movements that work on the upper back.
- Massage the affected area with oil and have a warm bath afterward.

Neck Pain

The neck is a common site of injury and pain. In yoga practitioners, especially those who practice inversions, this region needs careful attention. In headstand—an eagerly anticipated milestone in the practice of asanas—the weight of the body rests on the head and arms, placing the neck under a lot of stress. Headstand can aggravate existing neck problems or any scoliosis in the spine. Therefore, it is to be done only after careful, planned preparation of the neck and after checking for spinal asymmetry. The practice of shoulder stand too comes with these precautions, though the stress on the neck is less and of a slightly different nature.

In cases of neck pain or stiffness, we need to ask if there are any associated symptoms like giddiness and headache. The presence of such complaints will influence the choice of movements and body position.

A simple but useful point to remember is that neck movements for the correction of neck pain or stiffness are usually done together with arm movements. That is, whenever the head is raised, lowered, or rotated, the arms also move correspondingly. This ensures that we work not only on the neck but on the shoulders and upper back as well.

Deep twists like *ardha matsyendrasana* require that the person already possess considerable flexibility and strength in the neck. Therefore, such movements are of greater use for strengthening and prevention than in therapy. In therapy, simple twists in lying, seated, and standing positions are most commonly used.

Neck stiffness, especially in the elderly, requires gentle movements, with a restricted range of movement. In younger persons, more intense movements can be used.

Massage with oil, bathing in hot water, and avoiding direct exposure of the neck to cold air or water are all useful.

ASYMMETRY: SCOLIOSIS

Scoliosis is lateral deviation of the spine. As we discussed earlier, actively involving the spine in all movements is important in maximizing the effect of movements on the spine. However, the emphasis placed on such techniques must be in accordance with the person's capability, particularly in therapeutic situations. The practice of asymmetrical asanas is of great help in working with misalignments in the spine. Especially in children, during the period of growth, regular asana practice including appropriate asymmetrical movements can help to prevent the development of spinal misalignments and to correct existing ones. In adults, a complete cure may not be possible when the problem is the result of skeletal or other developmental disorders. However, asanas can help reduce the extent of the problem, thereby decreasing the symptoms and minimizing or relieving associated functional problems. We have seen cases where the deviation of the spine has resulted in dysfunction of organ systems, resulting in symptoms like tachycardia and occasional vomiting. These symptoms were relieved when the extent of the misalignment decreased with the regular practice of asanas. The wide range of movements available to us in asanas, especially asymmetrical movements combined with the emphasis on breathing, allows us to work with scoliosis very effectively. It also leaves us with the question of what movements and breathing to choose. The choice depends on several factors:

- The position of the misalignment in the spine
- The direction of the deviation
- The extent of the deviation
- Whether the scoliosis is accompanied by pain
- The presence of other symptoms
- The person's strength, flexibility, age, and general fitness

The following two case studies deal with scoliosis.

Case Study 6: Scoliosis

Prema was a fifty-seven-year-old housewife, five feet, three inches and 110 pounds. She had two grandchildren who kept her very busy. Her left ankle was twisted from birth, and she had undergone two surgeries to straighten her ankle and enable her to walk without using crutches. No movement was possible in her left ankle, which was still slightly twisted. Her left leg was also shorter than her right leg by approximately two inches. Consequently, she walked with a tilt to her left. Additionally, her right foot would swell if she remained standing for a long time.

I tested her spine and found that there was a deviation to the left in the lumbar region. Her back was strong, and she was able to do forward-bending movements quite well. Her upper back, however, was stiff. Her breathing was good. The difference in the length of her legs and the lack of movement in her left ankle had resulted in the scoliosis in her spine.

I did not choose standing asanas in her case for several reasons. First, standing would aggravate the swelling in her right leg. Second, she was on her feet for most of the day. Third, her natural standing position was already asymmetrical, with more weight placed on her right leg than her left. She had adapted to this over the decades. It would be difficult to work on each side individually in the standing position. In fact, in the initial stages, standing asanas could possibly even

Case Study 6: Scoliosis

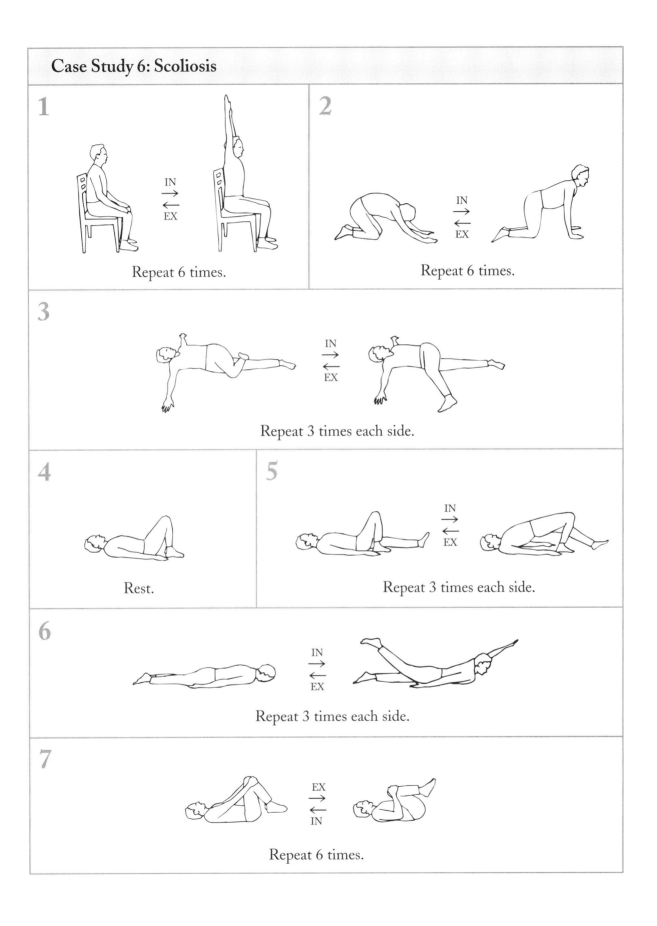

1

IN → ← EX

Repeat 6 times.

2

IN → ← EX

Repeat 6 times.

3

IN → ← EX

Repeat 3 times each side.

4

Rest.

5

IN → ← EX

Repeat 3 times each side.

6

IN → ← EX

Repeat 3 times each side.

7

EX → ← IN

Repeat 6 times.

increase the asymmetry. Finally, because the scoliosis was in her lower back, leg movements would probably be more effective in addressing it. In standing positions the legs would naturally be fixed.

She could not do inversions. This left a choice of seated and lying asanas. Lying asanas offered the greatest mobility and flexibility in working with her, and so the mainstay of her practice was asymmetrical movement from the lying position. Variations of *salabhasana*, *ardha salabhasana*, and *dvipadapitham* were very useful in her case. Lying twists were also useful. I developed the practice shown here by working with her for one month.

After a few months, the swelling in the right leg came down, and she also felt more energetic.

Case Study 7: Scoliosis

Paul was a very successful thirty-year-old businessman, five foot seven and 145 pounds. He was very disciplined in his daily routine and regularly practiced asanas for half an hour in the morning. He had scoliosis in his upper back and approached me for specific changes in his asana practice so that it would serve as a corrective exercise.

Paul was quite strong and flexible. However, he had been practicing mostly symmetrical asanas, including headstands and shoulder stands. To help correct his scoliosis, his practice needed to include asymmetrical forward and back bends and avoid inversions altogether. Headstands and shoulder stands

were not benefiting him. In fact, they could have been contributing to the scoliosis in his spine. He was comfortable with asymmetrical movements from the standing position because he was young and fit. I removed all inversions from his practice and instead introduced asymmetrical movements in both standing and lying positions. Holding after inhalation in backward-bending positions, especially asymmetrical ones, was very helpful in his case.

Case Study 7: Scoliosis
Key observations and assessment
• Fit young person with scoliosis of the upper spine.
Principal suggestions
• Include movements and stays in asymmetrical asanas.
• Emphasize arm movements in these asanas.
• Ensure that inhalation is emphasized in backward-bending asanas, and introduce holding after inhalation in these asanas.
• Avoid practicing inversions.

CONSTIPATION

In Ayurveda, movement is regarded as a quality of Vata, and hence most body functions involving movement are ascribed to Vata. Therefore, the function of bowel movement is attributed to one of the divisions of Vata, called apana vata. Apana vata is responsible for those functions involving expulsion of materials from the lower part of the body—for example, excretion and menstruation.

Regularizing the diet forms an important part of the approach to relieving constipation. In the face of an imbalanced and irregular diet, other measures may afford only

Case Study 7: Scoliosis

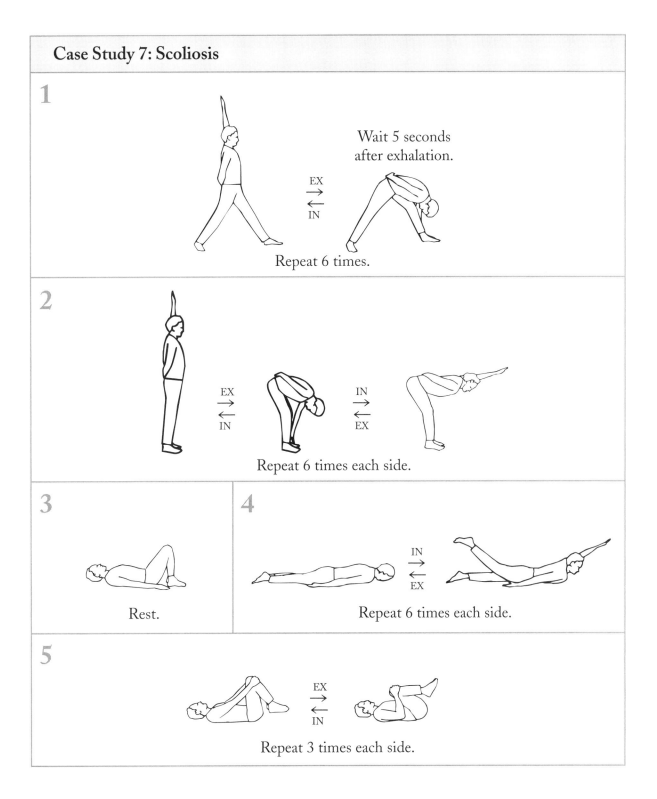

1

Wait 5 seconds after exhalation.

EX → ← IN

Repeat 6 times.

2

EX → ← IN

IN → ← EX

Repeat 6 times each side.

3

Rest.

4

IN → ← EX

Repeat 6 times each side.

5

EX → ← IN

Repeat 3 times each side.

temporary relief. Consideration of the agni also plays an important part in deciding on appropriate dietary changes. The presence of associated symptoms like headache may indicate specific imbalances of the agni. In such cases, adding appropriate herbs to the diet can be beneficial.

Ayurveda classifies bowel movement as a vega—a natural urge. Other examples of vegas are sneezing, coughing, thirst, hunger, and urination. To maintain health, Ayurveda suggests that these natural urges be neither suppressed nor initiated at will. Continued suppression or initiation of these can lead to irregularity in their natural occurrence. This is a possible contributing factor to be considered.

> **The vegas (natural urges) include:**
> • Urination
> • Bowel movement
> • Sneezing
> • Coughing
> • Hunger
> • Thirst

The mind too can play a major role in causing constipation. In fact, it is our mind that propels us to alter the natural timing of urges in our body when they interfere with our lifestyle or priorities. In addition, continued emotional disturbances like fear or the inability to mentally let go can also be important factors.

In the practice of asanas and pranayama, we aim to rectify the functioning of the apana vata through movements and breathing.

Exhalation works on the lower abdominal area and is also a process of elimination. Therefore, for constipation, we generally emphasize deep and long exhalation in asanas and pranayama. The use of exhalation also calms the person and helps in mentally letting go.

> **Important factors to consider in cases of constipation:**
> • Imbalanced diet.
> • Irregular timing of meals.
> • Suppression of natural urges.
> • Mental causes—an inability to let go or other emotional disturbances.

Case Study 8: Constipation

Rajkumar, a thirty-year-old medical representative, was five feet, nine inches and 140 pounds and had a cheerful personality. His job was quite demanding and required him to travel for at least two weeks each month. Rajkumar was able to cope with his work, though his wife felt that he was pushing himself too hard. He was healthy except for the irregular timing of his bowel movement; he often felt constipated and uneasy. The urge to empty his bowels occurred at unpredictable times during the day, especially after meals. The urge was overpowering and he found himself unable to resist it. The problem had been developing gradually over some time, but he had not attached much importance to it, as it had not interfered much with his lifestyle until now.

Rajkumar's appetite and digestion were

Case Study 8: Constipation

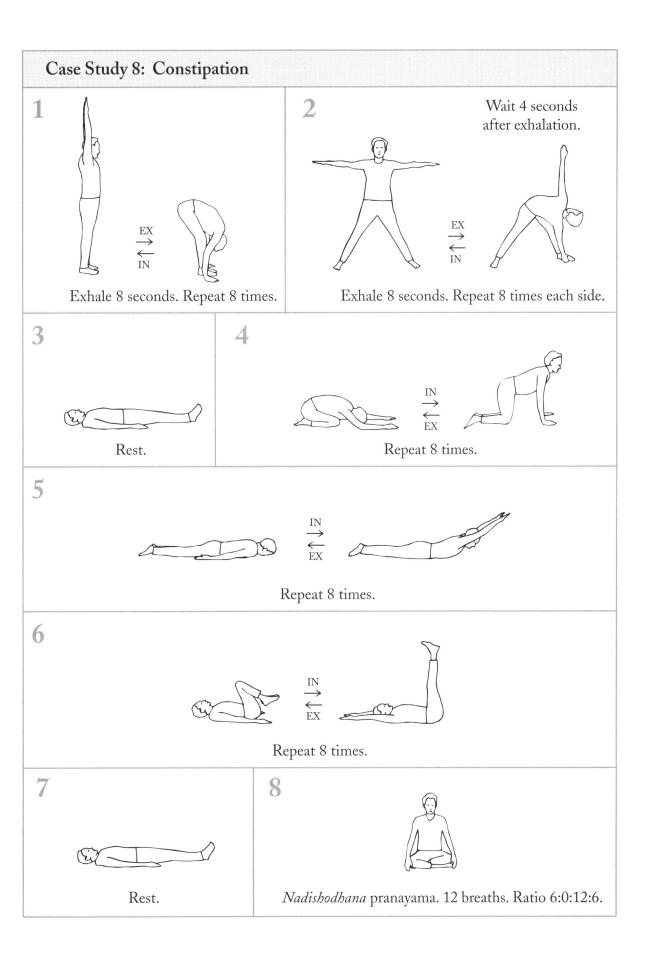

1

EX →
IN ←

Exhale 8 seconds. Repeat 8 times.

2

Wait 4 seconds after exhalation.

EX →
IN ←

Exhale 8 seconds. Repeat 8 times each side.

3

Rest.

4

IN →
EX ←

Repeat 8 times.

5

IN →
EX ←

Repeat 8 times.

6

IN →
EX ←

Repeat 8 times.

7

Rest.

8

Nadishodhana pranayama. 12 breaths. Ratio 6:0:12:6.

both good, and he was otherwise healthy. There did not appear to be any significant disturbance in the functioning of his agni. Despite his traveling and eating at many different places, he was quite conscious about his food intake, and therefore his diet was fairly balanced. But his mealtimes were irregular, and he usually had little food at dinner. On discussing his work and usual routine with him, I found that, in the past, he had habitually suppressed the natural urge to empty his bowels because of the demands of his work. His continued suppression of this natural urge could have upset its natural rhythm. In the absence of other major disturbances, it seemed that this interference with his natural urges (vegas) was an important factor contributing to the irregularity in his bowel movements.

Therefore, to gradually restore the natural timing of his bowel movement so that it would occur regularly in the mornings, I advised him to try to regularize his mealtimes and not ignore the natural rhythm of his body functions. I also suggested that he eat a better dinner and do the suggested asana and pranayama practice in the morning. He was able to devote about twenty-five minutes to his practice. As he was a fit young man, I designed a fairly active practice for him. Also, as the practice was to be done in the morning, raising his level of bodily activity would prepare him to face the day ahead. On observation I found that he was strong, but somewhat stiff, especially in his lower back. I started with simple asanas and breathing techniques, and when he was comfortable

with them, I introduced him about a month later to the practice shown here.

As he practiced the suggested asanas and pranayama in the morning, he found that they often stimulated the urge to have a bowel movement. Over a period of a few months, his bowel movement began to occur with increasing regularity and predictability in the mornings, without the need for the asana and pranayama practice to stimulate it.

Case Study 9: Constipation

Leela was a sixty-eight-year-old woman who had led a busy life. Apart from looking after her family, she had also been involved in many social activities. Over the previous year, she had reduced her activities and begun spending more time at home reading. She was of medium height and a little overweight. She had felt constipated with increasing frequency over the last year or so. She also had occasional pain in her joints, especially her knees. She felt that the pain increased whenever her bowel movement became more irregular.

It is a common observation that the natural aging process is accompanied by increasing dryness in the body and decreasing firmness and strength of body tissues. Dryness and lack of firmness are important properties of Vata. Ayurveda suggests that there is an impact from the qualities and functions of Vata in our bodies as we age. Common manifestations of this are some degree of constipation and restriction of mobility or pain in the joints, as in Leela's case. I suggested that she avoid or at least reduce the quantity of tubers

Case Study 9: Constipation

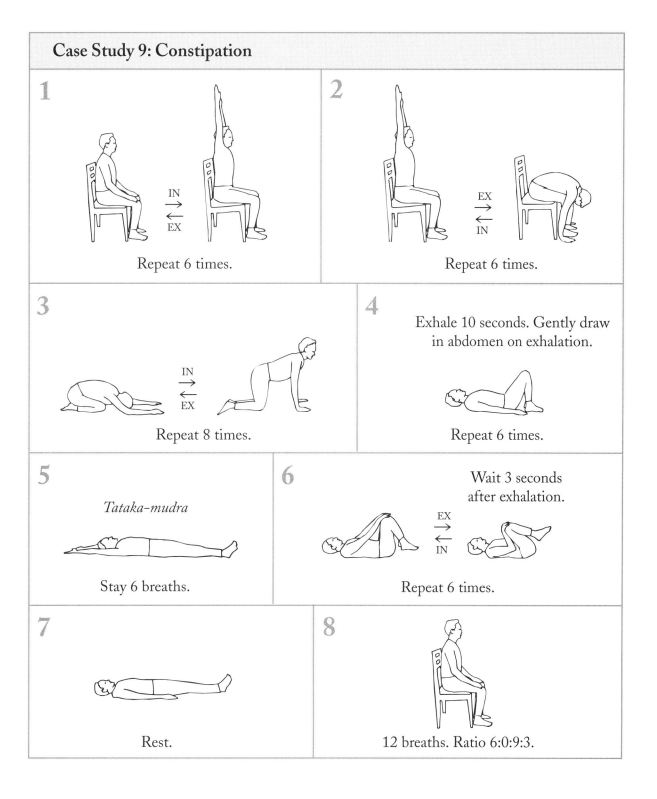

1

IN →
← EX

Repeat 6 times.

2

EX →
← IN

Repeat 6 times.

3

IN →
← EX

Repeat 8 times.

4

Exhale 10 seconds. Gently draw in abdomen on exhalation.

Repeat 6 times.

5

Tataka-mudra

Stay 6 breaths.

6

Wait 3 seconds after exhalation.

EX →
← IN

Repeat 6 times.

7

Rest.

8

12 breaths. Ratio 6:0:9:3.

and roots in her diet, particularly potatoes. I also advised her to eat more liquid foods like soups at night and to eat her food when it was hot or warm. Since coldness is a characteristic of Vata, warm food helps to reduce it. The warmth would also stimulate her digestion. Overall, her diet was to be light, as heavy food would be difficult for her to digest. Because of her reduced level of activity, she did not need to eat very much.

I designed the asana and pranayama practice, as in other cases of constipation, to emphasize exhalation. The duration of the practice was about thirty minutes. But compared to Rajkumar in case study 8, Leela was older and less fit. Therefore, the asanas I chose had to be much simpler, with no strenuous movements. Also, because of her joint pain, the practice had to avoid movements that would place stress on her joints, especially on her knees. Consequently, I included only seated or lying asanas. The practice of *tataka-mudra* was very useful in her case. It

helped to stimulate her lower abdomen and gradually tone her abdominal muscles. I introduced her to the practice over a period of two weeks.

In three months, her bowel movement became regular and more comfortable. She also lost a few pounds and felt more energetic.

Case Study 10: Constipation

Rajan, forty-four years old, was a senior executive. He told me he had constipation, which was associated with a feeling of discomfort and mild stomach pain at times. The discomfort and pain were relieved following his bowel movement but gradually returned later. He was of average height, with a slight paunch. He was not used to regular exercise, although lately he had been going for a walk three or four times a week. He said that he was fond of hot and spicy food, especially pickles.

Rajan was a classic example of how diet can be a cause of constipation. As I talked with him and found out the details of his diet, I realized that he was eating very spicy food at every meal. This excess of heating food in his diet was upsetting his agni. Reducing this dietary imbalance was the aim of the changes I suggested in his lifestyle. He was open to changes, and with his active participation I worked out a diet for him that contained less spice and more bitter and astringent foods. We also kept in mind that his food had to be fairly light and easy to digest. He had been eating a lot of yogurt, and on my advice he substituted it with buttermilk. He also avoided potatoes and pickles and included more cooked green

---

Case Study 9: Constipation
Key observations and assessment
• Elderly, overweight woman.
• Constipation associated with pain in joints.
Principal suggestions
• Diet
    Reduce consumption of roots and tubers, especially potatoes.
    Take warm liquid foods like soups at night.
• Asana
    Avoid movements that stress the knees.
    Use seated and lying asanas.
    Include *tataka-mudra*.
• Pranayama
    Ujjayi with suspension after exhalation.

vegetables. Instead of the deep-fried snacks he was used to having, he began to eat some fruit.

His asana practice was designed along the same general lines as the one I suggested to Rajkumar (see case study 8). But in Rajan's case, the practice of asanas and pranayama played a supporting role. Ayurveda was the key to correcting Rajan's problem. After changing his diet, he noticed a significant improvement in a little over a month. His stomachache and discomfort virtually disappeared, and his bowel movement was much easier and more frequent. However, he found that when he was careless with his diet, the problem sometimes recurred.

MENSTRUAL PROBLEMS

Just as apana vata plays a role in the elimination process, it is responsible for menstruation too. Normally, the functions of apana vata occur with regularity. Just as bowel movement once or twice a day and urination six or more times a day are normal, menstruation at an interval of about twenty-five to thirty days is normal. This regularity of function is a significant feature of the undisturbed functioning of apana vata. Apart from apana vata, the level of heat in the system is another important factor in ensuring the proper occurrence of the menstrual cycle.

The diet and the mind can influence the cycle. The functioning of apana vata is bound to our mental state. When we are anxious—for example, before an important examination—our mind stimulates apana vata, and we often feel the urge to empty our bladder. As urination is a partly voluntary function, we are able to appreciate the connection here clearly. The same connection is also present but less obvious in the menstrual cycle. Therefore, psychological disturbances must be considered as possible important contributors to irregularities in menstruation.

> **Important factors to consider in cases of menstrual problems:**
> - Functioning of apana vata.
> - Level of heat in the system.
> - Psychological or emotional disturbances.
> - Dietary imbalances.

Case Study 11: Menstrual Problems

Nineteen-year-old Rohini, born and brought up in Chennai, India, went to the east coast of the United States for college. She was very happy to be admitted to the university of her choice and was enthusiastic about her studies. All was well in her life, except that she stopped menstruating shortly after arriving in the United States, and this absence of menstruation persisted for an entire year. At the end of the year, when she returned to India to visit her family, her worried mother sought my help.

Rohini did not consider the disturbance in her menstrual cycle to be a serious problem. Rohini had started menstruating at the age of fourteen, but her periods were somewhat irregular for the first two years. During that time, her periods would occur once every three or four months, but the flow was normal, for a duration of three days, with no pain or cramps. Subsequently, her periods began to occur regularly, until she left India.

She was a vegetarian and was used to eating spicy foods at home. After moving to the United States, she had been taking more salads, fruits, and juices. She had to study a lot and did not have much time for exercise or outdoor activities.

Rohini's constitution was basically dominated by qualities of Kapha. Apart from the disturbance in her menstruation, she was healthy. Her digestion was good and she slept well, but her lifestyle in the United States was reducing the heat in her system. The cold climate, cold and raw food, lack of spices in her diet, and lack of exercise were all contributing to the lack of heat—the principal quality of Pitta.

I advised her to include more solids in her food and to cook them with some spices like red pepper and ginger and to include some lemon. I also suggested that she consume warm, cooked vegetables in place of salads and more hot soups than cold juices. I also suggested two Ayurvedic medicines, one to induce the menstrual cycle and the other to regularize the flow of Vata.

She was quite strong and flexible and her breath was good. Since exercise was important for her, the practice I designed for her was active.

Rohini followed these suggestions when she returned to the United States. Her menstrual cycle resumed in two months, and the subsequent cycles were regular. She discontinued the medicines but adhered to the diet changes and had no further problems.

Case Study 11: Menstrual problems

Key observations and assessment
- Young woman, absence of menstruation in the last year.
- Likely to be related to decrease in level of heat in the system due to dietary and environmental changes.

Principal suggestions
- Diet
    Take more solid food, cooked with pepper, ginger, and lemon.
    Take more cooked vegetables, hot porridges, and soups.
- Asana
    Asana practice leading to shoulder stand.
    Include asymmetrical standing asanas.
    Ensure exhalation is long. Include suspension after exhalation.

Case Study 12: Menstrual Problems

Mala, thirty-five years old, was the mother of two school-age children. She ran a boutique. In the last year, her menstrual cycle had become shorter, with her periods occurring every twenty days. This sapped her energy and she felt unable to cope with her work and family. She had a medical checkup, but there was no detectable underlying pathology. She was of average build and appeared worried and tired.

Mala began menstruating at the age of twelve and had a fairly regular cycle until now. In her early years, she occasionally suffered from cramps, but this problem did not occur later. Her flow was quite heavy for three days and subsided gradually by the fifth day. She had been very busy in the last year in setting up her boutique. She enjoyed running the boutique, but with her family responsibilities also taking up much of her time, she had hardly any time to relax. As a result, she was feeling irritable and pressed. Her husband was quite supportive of her initiatives, but he was equally busy with his job. Mala was quite fond of spicy food, and her diet did not include much in the way of fresh fruits and vegetables. She had at least three cups of strong coffee every day and was often constipated. She had been in the habit of taking a walk in the evenings, but now, after starting the boutique, she was unable to find the time for it.

Mala's constitution was dominated by Pitta. She also seemed quite restless by nature. She had set some goals for herself in her business and was anxious to reach them. She looked at her health problems as hurdles in the path to these goals. She was seeking a quick remedy to her problem so that she could carry on with her work.

Her mind was playing a major role in creating her health problems. Nevertheless, her food habits could not be ignored. To start with, I suggested that she restrict her intake of coffee to two cups a day. Her breakfast was to be light, probably warm porridge with some fruit. For both lunch and dinner I advised her to cut back on spices and try to eat more green vegetables. She also promised that she would have her meals at regular times and not go long periods without eating.

Since her mind was the driving force behind her lifestyle disturbances, a change in her mental outlook would help sustain other changes. Therefore, I designed an asana and pranayama program for her that would relax her, reduce her stress, and help her view her lifestyle from a fresh perspective.

She was ready to devote half an hour in the morning to her asana practice and meditation. She had faith in the Divine, and I suggested a mantra in accordance with her belief to help her calm down. Her asana practice was twenty minutes long, with an emphasis on exhalation. She started her practice with twelve breaths of shitali pranayama. At the end of her asana practice, she again did twelve breaths of shitali pranayama and followed this with twelve breaths of nadishodhana pranayama. In the evening, before dinner, she practiced relaxation breathing for ten minutes, lying on her back with her legs resting on a stool (fig. 8.11).

After three months, Mala reported that her menstrual cycle had reverted to twenty-eight days and that she was feeling much more relaxed. She was getting help from one of her friends in running the boutique and

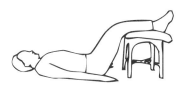

24 breaths, with mantra.

Fig. 8.11. Case Study 12: The most important component of the practice was the extended exhalation, done with an appropriate mantra.

Case Study 12: Menstrual Problems

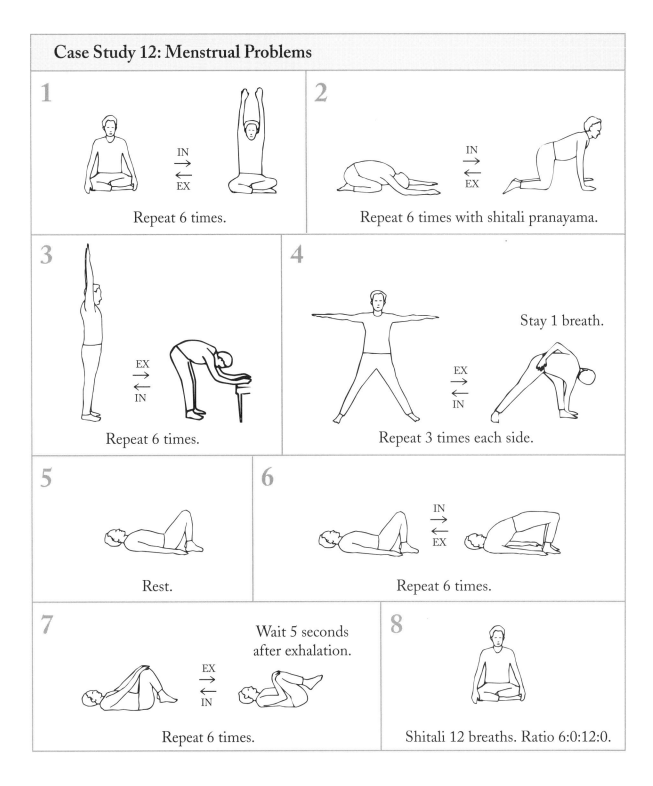

1 Repeat 6 times.

2 Repeat 6 times with shitali pranayama.

3 Repeat 6 times.

4 Stay 1 breath. Repeat 3 times each side.

5 Rest.

6 Repeat 6 times.

7 Wait 5 seconds after exhalation. Repeat 6 times.

8 Shitali 12 breaths. Ratio 6:0:12:0.

consequently had more time for herself at home. Her bowel movement was now regular, and she felt lighter and energetic.

Case Study 12: Menstrual problems
Key observations and assessment
- 35-year-old mother of two children. Increased frequency of menstruation and heavier flow.
- Restless nature, pressures herself to achieve business goals and take care of family simultaneously.

Principal suggestions
- Yoga program
    20-minute program with emphasis on exhalation. Begin and end with shitali pranayama, with mantra.
    Emphasize relaxation breathing with mantra.
- Diet
    Fewer spices in food. More fruits and vegetables. Reduce coffee intake.

Case Study 13: Menstrual Problems

Uma, thirty-seven years old, was a housewife with two school-age children. Her periods had been irregular for about a year. The cycle was unpredictable, ranging from twenty-five to forty days. Her husband's job involved much travel, and so she was in complete charge of the household. She was also an active member of a ladies' club, looking after the accounts and organizing several activities. She was tall and lean. Her constitution was characteristically Vata. She was generally constipated but had not taken this seriously. However, I found that she was quite concerned about her health. She was somewhat impatient when answering questions, and she herself confessed that she was the type of person who liked to be involved in everything.

She also told me that she did not sleep very well at night.

Her diet included fruit but few green vegetables. She was fond of fried foods and had such snacks frequently. She was quite strong but had stiff hamstrings and her breathing was shallow.

This was a clear case of a disturbance of apana vata. Her constitution was dominated by Vata, and the constipation was indicative of the malfunctioning of apana vata. Mentally, her need to be active all the time—the feeling that she had to be "doing something"—was contributing to the problem. It was important for her to relax and reduce her level of constant mental activity.

I suggested an asana practice for twenty minutes with emphasis on extended exhalation. The practice ended with twenty-four breaths of *anuloma* ujjayi pranayama (1:2 ratio), followed by meditation for fifteen minutes. She had attended some yoga classes a few years ago and was familiar with some of the movements. This made it easier for her to do the asana practice. I also asked her to have an oil massage once a week.

For Reflection

When dealing with problems with the menstrual cycle, as well as with constipation, the problem-specific guidelines to be followed in designing an asana practice are not very different. In both cases we emphasize exhalation and seek to remove the complicating mental factors, commonly an inability to relax or let go. If the disturbance in the apana is due to

Pitta, the food and pranayama have to be changed accordingly. The true individuality of the practice lies in the observation of the person and the personalization of the practice for that individual. The similarity stems from the basis in Ayurveda—in both situations we are trying to rectify a problem associated with apana vata.

This is a conceptualized relationship that Ayurveda postulates between body functions such as menstruation, defecation, urination, and so on. It is not possible either to see apana vata physically or to manipulate it directly. But it is useful as an approach to therapy, especially in a noninvasive system such as yoga.

ASTHMA

Although it is not possible to explain the approach of yoga and Ayurveda to functional problems in detail here, we include an outline of the approach to one major disorder—asthma—as an example.

Ayurvedic Factors

The *Caraka-Samhita*, one of the most important texts in Ayurveda, lists the following ten factors to be considered in the treatment of any disease. All these must be kept in mind:

- The strength of the agni
- The person's overall strength
- The dhatu that is affected
- The person's constitution
- What food the person is used to
- The person's habits and lifestyle
- The place where the person was born
- The person's mind and mental state
- The person's age
- The time of year

Food Guidelines

In cases of asthma, food guidelines based on the six tastes are as follows:

- Sweet: Fruits can be taken but avoid artificial sweets.
- Bitter: can be taken
- Astringent: can be included, except those based on dairy products
- Pungent: can be taken if mixed with other products
- Sour: Tamarind, lime, and so on must be reduced or avoided, but bread is alright.
- Salt: should be reduced

There are also several general food guidelines. In general, asthmatics should reduce or avoid the following specific types of food:

- Dairy products, especially cheese
- Salty, fatty, and fried food
- Sour items from natural sources like tamarind, lime, orange, and so on
- Raw food
- Cold drinks

One should eat light, warm, cooked food. In general, one third of the food intake at every meal must be liquid. Dinner must be very light, consisting mostly of liquids. These general food guidelines can vary based on the specific dosha out of balance.

Numerous diet and lifestyle changes and herbs are outlined in Ayurveda for the management of asthma. Several of them can be usefully applied in many cases.

Asana Guidelines

There are several general guidelines for designing an asana program for asthma. In general, asthmatics should do the following:

- Exercise within limits (excessive exercise can trigger an asthma attack, but too little exercise will not be beneficial).
- Ascertain these limits through observation of the breath and taking the pulse.
- Allow adequate rest between postures.
- Encourage diaphragmatic breathing.
- Choose suitable postures (inverted postures are more for prevention than cure; though they can be introduced to young asthmatics, inverted positions should only be taught to others when they are fit enough to do them).

Breathing and Pranayama Guidelines

In asthma, the airways are obstructed and the person has difficulty breathing, especially exhaling. This is usually reflected in pulmonary function tests as a decrease in the expiratory flow rate. Many asthmatics commonly have an exhalation of extended duration. It is in rapid exhalation that their capacity is limited. Therefore, when possible, emphasis on rapid exhalation is the best approach in designing a yoga practice for asthma.

It is with this in mind that classical yoga texts like the *Hatha-Yoga-Pradipika* suggest fast bellows breathing through the nostrils (kapalabhati pranayama) for asthma. This is, of course, not to be applied indiscriminately. Kapalabhati pranayama is a fairly strenuous practice; not everyone can do it in its classical form. But the principle is sound—it only needs to be modified to suit the individual's capacity.

Stepped exhalation (exhaling for a few seconds, pausing for a few seconds, exhaling again and pausing, and so on) is not advisable. Stepped exhalation amounts to retaining the air in the lungs for a longer time than normal. It is similar to holding the breath after inhalation. This is not helpful in asthma, where hyperinflation of the lungs is already a possible consequence of the disease process.

From the Ayurvedic viewpoint, asthma is usually associated with an imbalance of the qualities and functions of the Kapha dosha, and therefore kapalabhati pranayama is especially suitable. However, this may not always be the best choice. The pranayama must be chosen and modified intelligently depending on the person and the involvement of other doshas. See the guidelines outlined in chapter 6.

Sound

Sound can help to promote complete exhalation and therefore can be used gainfully in asthma. Ideally, the sound used must be full throated, done in seated or standing positions or in forward-bending movements. The pitch must be comfortable for the person; this can be varied as the person progresses. Humming is generally not a good idea, as it can irritate the throat and result in coughing. It can also leave the person with a restricted feeling, unlike fully vocalized sounds, which usually promote a feeling of openness and lightness.

Sequences for Practice

SVASTHA STHIRA-SUKHA *SERIES*

In this book we have emphasized that correct practice of asanas gives us strength, flexibility, structural alignment, proper functioning of body systems, and mental steadiness. To work toward these five goals simultaneously in a balanced manner, we have designed the sequences in this appendix. These sequences, which progress from simple to difficult, combine movement in all three axes and incorporate dynamic movements in a flowing series. To derive the best from asana practice remember that it is essential to pay attention, to your breath and to make sure that your mind does not wander. Work in as you work out.

Guidelines

1. These sequences are designed for healthy adults.
2. Do not force your body or breath. Rest when required.
3. Increase the number of repetitions gradually.
4. Repeat asymmetrical asanas on both sides.
5. As you progress you can introduce holding postures and suspending the breath.
6. Difficult asanas should be attempted only after you are comfortable doing series like the ones in this appendix.

Practice sequence 1: Repeat all steps 3 times

1

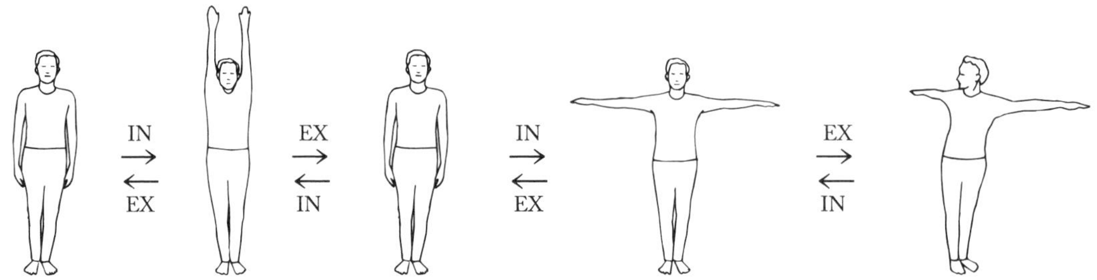

IN → ← EX   EX → ← IN   IN → ← EX   EX → ← IN

2

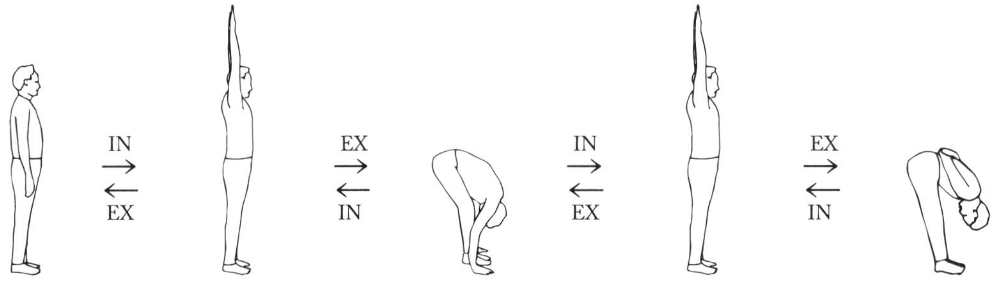

IN → EX   EX → IN   IN → EX   EX → IN

3

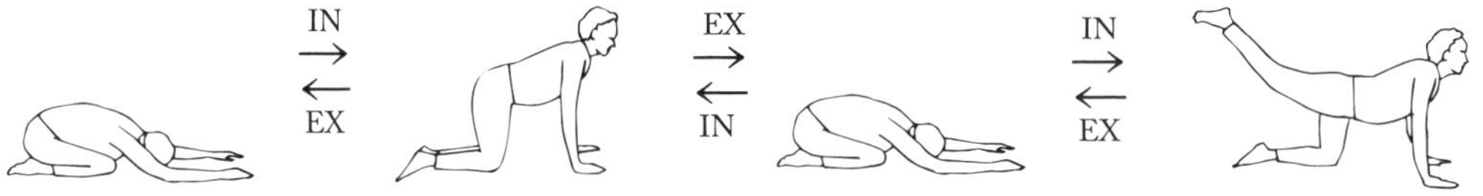

IN → ← EX   EX → ← IN   IN → ← EX

REST

4

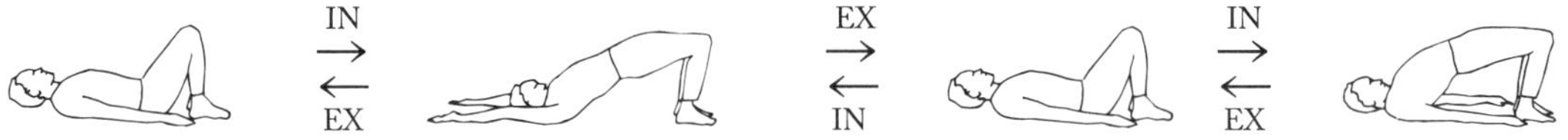

IN → ← EX   EX → ← IN   IN → ← EX

5

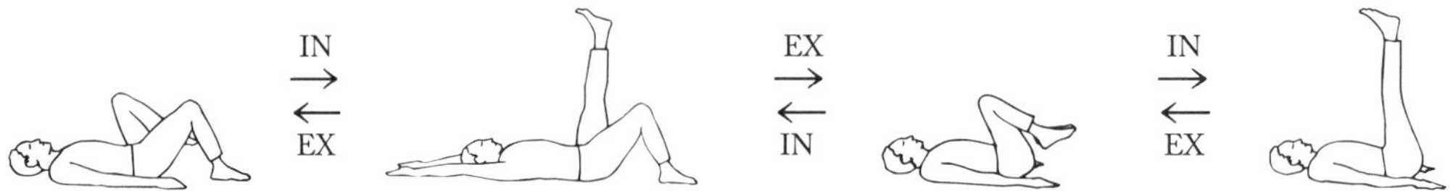

IN → ← EX   EX → ← IN   IN → ← EX

REST

Practice sequence 1 (continued) : Repeat all steps 3 times

6

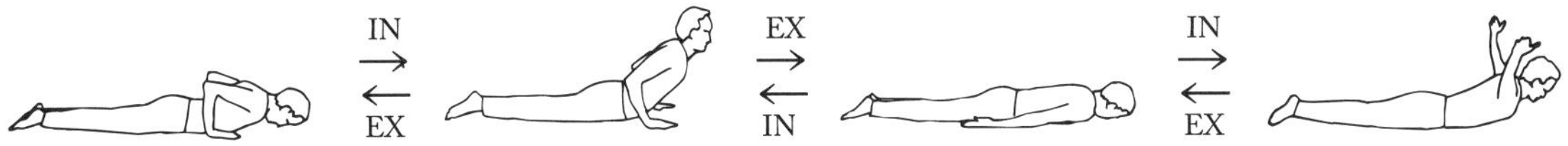

IN → / EX ←   EX → / IN ←   IN → / EX ←

7

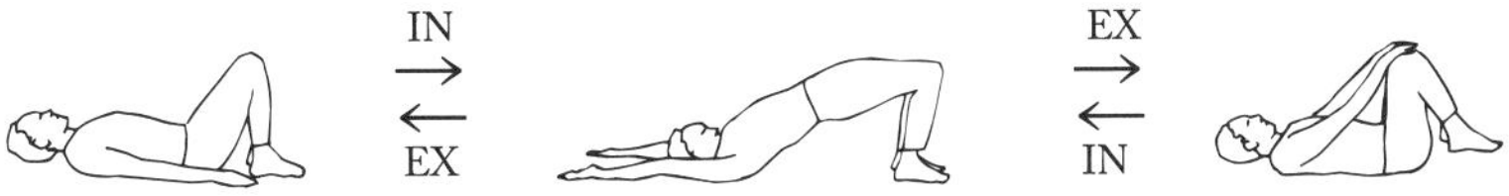

IN → / EX ←   EX → / IN ←

REST

8

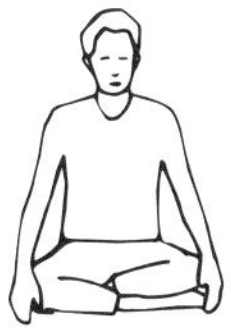

12 breaths — *ujjayi* pranayama — long exhalation

Practice sequence 2: Repeat all steps 3 times

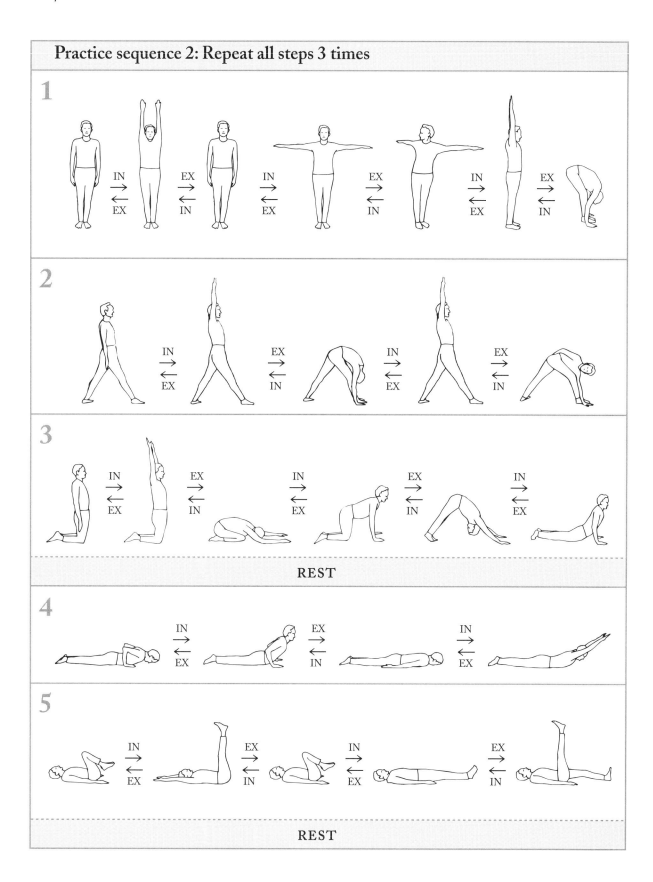

Practice sequence 2 (continued): Repeat all steps 3 times

6

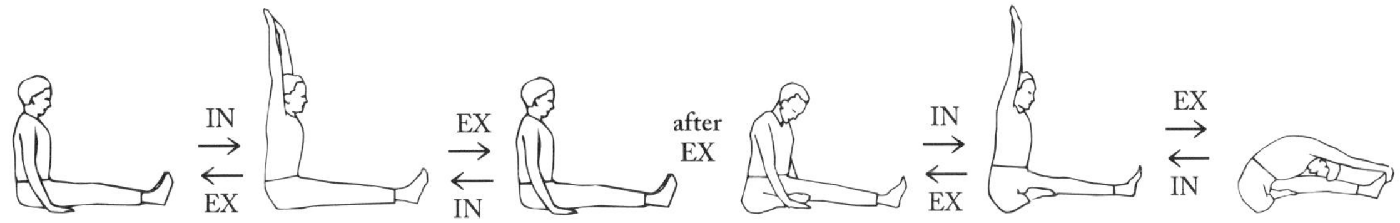

IN → ← EX   EX → ← IN   after EX   IN → ← EX   EX → ← IN

REST

7

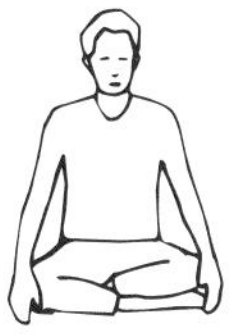

12 breaths — *anuloma ujjayi* pranayama — long exhalation

Practice sequence 3: Repeat all steps 3 times

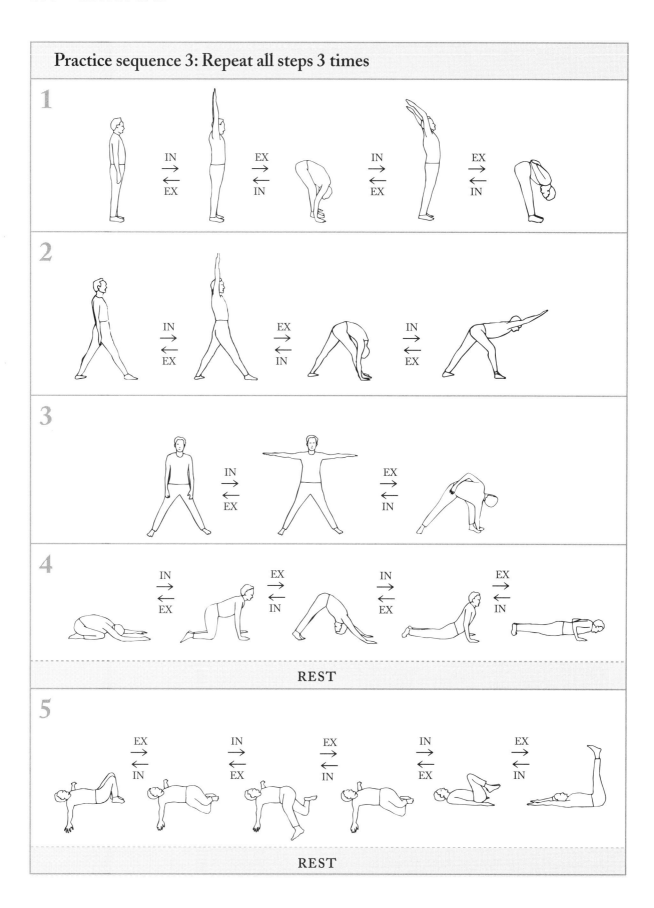

REST

REST

Practice sequence 3 (continued): Repeat all steps 3 times

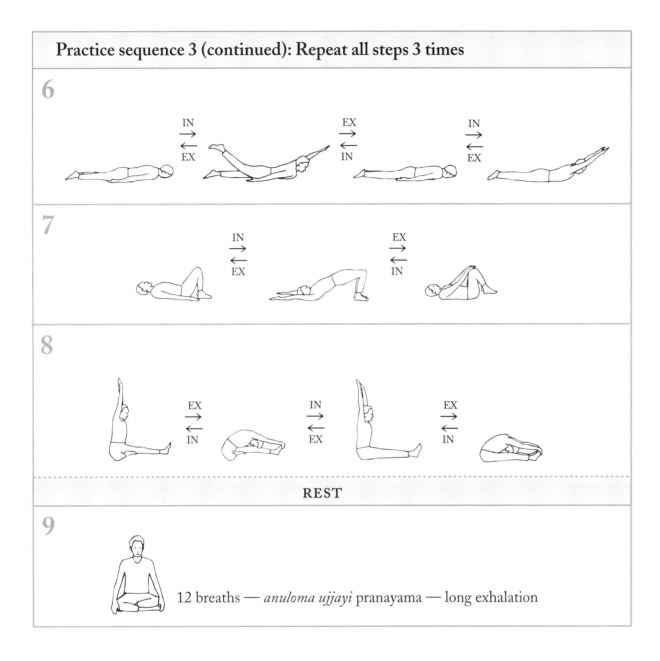

6

7

8

REST

9

12 breaths — *anuloma ujjayi* pranayama — long exhalation

Practical Considerations in Pranayama

PRANAYAMA IS complex. As you practice, questions and problems relating to your body, breathing, and concentration will arise. It is important to resolve them if you are to refine and develop your practice. Below we give a list of practical questions for consideration. If you find that any of the questions are relevant to you—and it is likely that you will—you should discuss them with your yoga teacher. If you are a yoga teacher, the questions below can help you evaluate and deepen your understanding of pranayama.

DEFINING PRANAYAMA

Pranayama is defined as consciously changing the pattern of breathing. Running, singing, and chanting are all conscious activities that change the pattern of breathing. Would they qualify as pranayama? Why or why not? What qualities distinguish pranayama from these activities? Can some of these activities be modified to derive benefits similar to those obtained by the practice of pranayama? If so, how?

PASSIVE OBSERVATION OF THE BREATH

We said that passive observation of the breath can be used to focus the mind. What criteria can be used to determine if passive observation or active regulation would be more appropriate for a person?

PREPARATION FOR PRANAYAMA

1. Is kapalabhati pranayama necessary to prepare the breath for the practice of pranayama? Why or why not?

2. Pranayama involves staying in a position and breathing. Therefore, when using asanas as a preparation for pranayama, is it better to emphasize staying in asanas and breathing rather than making dynamic movements?

3. As a preparation for pranayama, is it better to do asanas with active jumping movements as a continuous series, or is it better to use the individual asanas in a sequence?

POSTURE FOR PRANAYAMA

1. A person has difficulty in doing *utkatasana* and *dvipadapitham*. He can do *vajrasana*, *uttanasana*, *parsva uttanasana*, and *pascimatanasana*. What posture would you choose for him to do pranayama in? Why?

2. A fit thirty-year-old man wants to do pranayama with a ratio of 15:0:15:0. What postures would you use in his asana practice to prepare for the pranayama practice? If the same person wants to do pranayama with a ratio of 12:0:24:0, what postures would you suggest?

BREATHING IN PRANAYAMA

1. Jane, thirty years old, has difficulty exhaling smoothly. The flow and method of her breathing need correction. Would you choose a seated or lying position for observa-

tion and correction? Why? What instructions would you give her?

2. Mary experienced depression due to a personal loss. Is it advisable to teach her breathing emphasizing the chest with a ratio of 1:0:1:0? On what criteria would you base your assessment of her progress?

3. Gail is often afraid. A yoga teacher taught her breathing emphasizing the chest with a ratio of 1:0:1:0. She does not feel comfortable with it. What could the reason be? What would you do to help her?

4. John is used to doing meditation in the seated position for two hours every day. When he started practicing pranayama, he felt dizzy when he tried to increase the length of his inhalation. What could be the reason for this? What would you do?

5. Exhalation is normally a passive process of which we are not conscious. That is, if it were not for our conscious intervention, the air would have left our lungs without our being aware of it. Does that mean that conscious extension of exhalation is a retention of air?

6. Which of the following will increase the rajasic tendency of the mind: forced inhalation or forced exhalation?

7. Kapalabhati and *Bhastrika* both involve fast abdominal breathing. The breath is neither long and steady nor smooth and subtle. Therefore, they do not seem to come under pranayama according to the definition in the *Yoga-Sutras* (2.50). Why do we classify them under pranayama? What is their use?

8. After practicing pranayama in *Brahmasana* for 15 minutes, Mary feels tension in

her neck and pain in her knees and middle back. Suggest a suitable 10-minute asana practice to be practiced after pranayama.

9. At the end of inhalation, instead of allowing the abdomen to move out a little, John tends to draw it in a little, thus forcing the diaphragm upward. Why does this need correction? How would you correct it?

10. John feels that the use of ratios in pranayama is a distraction. Is it true?

11. Gail feels that her mind wanders if she does slow, deep breathing without ratios, whereas Mary feels that her mind wanders when she does use ratios. Consider the possible differences in their mental dispositions.

12. Is there more scope for observation of the breath when pranayama is done without using ratios?

Mantra in Pranayama

1. If we use a mantra during the practice of pranayama, how can we watch our breath? Won't it be distracting?

2. Is it essential to know the meaning of the mantra before using it?

3. How do I choose a mantra based on my own religion? Will I get the same benefit?

4. It is possible that in olden days, there was no accurate method of time measurement (no clocks!). Maybe that is why a mantra was used. Isn't it enough to simply use a clock to time the ratios during pranayama practice? Why use a mantra?

5. John says that counting the number of his breaths during pranayama is distracting. Instead, he sets a clock for fifteen minutes. Which is the better method? Why?

6. What is the difference between doing pranayama with a ratio 4:0:8:0 for 48 breaths, and 8:0:16:0 for 24 breaths? Note that both work out to the same total time.

7. How will you decide when a person is ready to practice all the three bandhas?

8. Should we do pranayama with eyes open or eyes closed? Why? In what circumstances would you suggest keeping the eyes open?

9. John has a deviated nasal septum. One of his nostrils is partially blocked most of the time. He gets a headache after nadi-shodhana pranayama. What would you advise him to do?

10. Martha, in spite of practicing asanas, yawns frequently. What type of pranayama would you advise her to do?

11. Before teaching stepped breathing in pranayama, what is the most important observation to be made?

Interview with A. G. Mohan

Q. YOU HAVE SPOKEN of clarity and rationality in the preface of this book. Why are they relevant? What is clear and rational in the field of yoga?

A. The current explosion in the popularity of yoga, while valuable in that it has brought some of its benefits to a large number of people, has come at a price. Questioning has taken a backseat to adherence to lineage and tradition, resulting in great confusion in the field of yoga. This situation is not a reflection on the yoga teachers in the West, most of whom display much commitment and sincerity in learning, practicing, and teaching yoga. It has resulted largely because the yoga teachers in the West are not offered proper tools, or access to question the views of their teachers. This is particularly counterproductive in these times. It is now necessary to be critical of conflicting presentations in the field of yoga and make a sound choice

Put simply, a rational view comes from a logical theory that is supported by observation. This applies to yoga as to any field. It is important to keep in mind that when there is a conflict between rationality and a source quoted as being authentic, more weight must be attached to rationality in most circumstances. This is because an approach based on suspect rationality is much less likely to yield expected results than one with sound rationality backing it, regardless of the source.

The only undeniably authentic and rational text on yoga is the *Yoga-Sutras* of Patanjali. There are at least ten published commentaries and subcommentaries on this text, in Sanskrit, currently available. It was customary for these commentators to question their own statements and provide answers.

The point here is that in the past blind adherence to tradition was not demanded of the student in the study of yoga. Likewise, today's yoga students must be offered the proper tools for inquiry, as well as the right to question the views of their teachers. It is important to bear in mind that the future of yoga is not served when teachers advocate methods that will not stand up to unbiased scrutiny. Popularity is not a substitute for evidence, and faith is not a substitute for sound method.

Q. You made a statement in the book that the benefits of the postures are usually greatly exaggerated in ancient yoga texts, for example, that several asanas are able to cure all diseases. Can you expand on this? Are you saying that the ancient texts are not a reliable or accurate guide to asanas? How can you contradict the ancient texts on yoga?

A. The *Yoga-Sutras* are the defining text on yoga, and they do not deal with the practice of asanas in any significant detail. Therefore, when speaking of asanas in ancient yoga texts, I am not contradicting the *Yoga-Sutras*.

There are several other texts on yoga, like the *Yoga-Yajnavalkya*, *Hatha-Yoga-Pradipika*, *Shiva-Samhita*, *Gheranda-Samhita*, and the Yoga Upanishads. They contain descriptions of asanas—not the method of doing them, but simply the body positions. The descriptions are very similar across texts and it possible that some of them are borrowed verses from the *Yoga-Yajnavalkya*, which is thought to be the oldest of these texts (and is also the most organized of them).

One important reason for the confusion surrounding these other yoga texts is their mixed content: They contain everything from tantric sex practices and cutting the frenulum of the tongue, to useful guidelines on pranayama and standard descriptions borrowed from nondualistic philosophy. This simply reflects their varied sources and the wide scope of the information, ideology, and beliefs included in these texts.

The point I am trying to drive home is that these yoga texts are not like the *Yoga-Sutras*, in which every word is chosen with care and precision. They are to be interpreted cautiously, not taken literally.

Q. You studied for many years under Sri T. Krishnamacharya, who was undeniably an authentic teacher of yoga. Did he ever write anything on these ancient yoga texts?

A. Sri Krishnamacharya wrote a book called the *Yoga Makaranda* in 1934. The book, his wife has said, was written in just two days at the request of the King of Mysore (one of the kingdoms then existing in southern India). This book has long been out of print, but copies of this book are still available in libraries.

The first half of this book discusses a wide variety of topics ranging from the mudras and *kriya*s (cleansing techniques) to meditation, all presented largely as is from the ancient yoga texts. The second half of this book deals with the practice of asanas. The descriptions of the ideal form of the asanas, along with lists of conditions that the asanas are useful for treating, are also mostly presented as in the ancient yoga texts.

Many of these practices like the kriyas were not advocated by Sri Krishnamacharya. During my studies with him in his later years he pointed out that some of these practices could be harmful and others were inapplicable in the context of modern lifestyle.

However, some significant features of this book areas follows:

- The book details a step-by-step sequential approach to many asanas, accompanied by photographs. You can see that many of the sequences are a simpler version of some of the sequences taught now as *ashtangayoga*.
- It emphasizes the importance of breathing and clearly describes the breathing patterns to be followed.
- It does not propose a therapy based on cakra theory, but instead uses Ayurvedic terminology to describe diseases, just as the old yoga texts did.

There is also a video of Sri T. Krishnamacharya doing asanas, filmed in the 1930s. It was included as part of a video on his centenary celebration called "One Hundred Years of Beatitude," produced by CNRS Audiovisuel in France. I was the convenor of his centenary celebration. In this video you can see him demonstrate the principles of movement in all three axes.

Q. In summary, how would you suggest that an approach to asanas be judged?

A. The validity of an approach to asanas is not to be judged by rigid adherence to the form of the posture as described in assorted yoga texts, but by the method of doing them—most important, whether that method makes sense. It is only logical that we should adopt a structured, progressive, and personalized approach, not just in asana practice but in any form of exercise or therapy. In fact, if you choose to reject such an approach, it follows that you should ask yourself if your asana practice is sound and if so, on what basis.

Q. Yoga therapy is gaining in popularity and acceptance. What is the basis for yoga therapy in the ancient texts?

A. This is a question that is gaining importance. Regarding the foundations of yoga therapy, it is essential that you be aware that there is little in the way of a separate yoga physiology on which to base treatment. As we have said, the yoga texts describe diseases using terminology borrowed from Ayurveda. They only add general references to the "flow of prana," which should be understood as indicating the proper functioning of that body part. There is no technique possible to feel or see the flow of prana, or manipulate it like a physical entity. When yoga texts like the *Yoga-Yajnavalkya* speak of focusing the prana somewhere, it is not during the practice of asanas but during the practice of pranayama, and even then it means only the focusing of the mind.

In Ayurveda, the three-dosha theory is used practically everywhere as an approach to understanding physical health and disease, and the three gunas as an approach to mental health and disease. This can be verified by simply browsing through any translation of any major text on Ayurveda.

Q. Can we base yoga therapy on the cakra model?

A. In classical texts on tantra that speak of the cakras in detail, the cakras are conceptualized as "knots of bondage." The path is usually presented as piercing, opening, dissolving, or untying each cakra in turn, which essentially means transcending the mental constructs binding you to that aspect of your existence and thereby moving one step closer to freedom. The methods suggested are mostly centered on meditation in a seated position. They do not suggest methods for treatment of physical disease. Nor do the yoga texts link the cakras to specific diseases. Furthermore, there is no mention of the cakras as a basis for diagnosis or treatment in the ancient texts on Ayurveda.

The cakras are linked to the five forms of matter and emotions, but this is a method of meditation and eventually transcendence, and not a therapy. If there is a sound basis for linking specific diseases, using contemporary medical terminology, to the "misalignment" of particular cakras, I would like to know what it is.

Q. What about treatment based on the five *koshas*?

A. The five *koshas* or "sheaths" (*annamaya, pranamaya, manomaya, vijnanamaya,* and *anandamaya*) are not linked to the treatment of disease, either in the yoga texts, ayurveda or the *Taittiriya-Upanishad* (in which the five *koshas* are detailed).

The *Taittiriya-Upanishad* is a presentation of the psychology behind the path to freedom and fulfillment. There are commentaries on it written by many extraordinary luminaries of ancient India, like Sankara and Vidyaranya. It complements the psychology of the *Yoga-Sutras* elegantly and is quoted in commentaries on the *Yoga-Sutras*. The *Taittiriya-Upanishad* does not present a method of therapy. The practices mentioned under all the *koshas* are meditative practices. There is no practice under the *anandamaya kosha*—rather, it is the description of the experience that results. This point is stated by Sankara in his commentary.

Q. How do you link diseases as explained in modern medicine with the terms used in Ayurveda?

A. It is not easy to link ancient and modern medical systems. Diabetes, for example, is usually compared with *prameha* or *madhumeha*, conditions when the urine output is increased or the urine is sweet. These are symptoms of uncontrolled diabetes. However, an increase in quantity and frequency of urine output can also be seen in disorders of the urinary system and in other body systems as well. It is important not to draw direct correlations between Ayurvedic terms and modern disease descriptions on the basis of single symptoms. Furthermore, Ayurvedic concepts like the doshas should be considered conceptual and not physical entities.

Q. You have not spoken about sound and chanting in this book. Aren't they useful tools in yoga therapy?

A. Sound is certainly useful in yoga therapy. However, we have spoken little of the use of sound or chanting in this book—and with good reason. They need to be dealt with separately in detail because, in the areas of sound and chanting, there is thorough analysis and extensive literature available in classical Vedic literature on phonetics. The effect of pitch and other characteristics of chanting on the mind and the reasons why it should be done in a certain way have all been explained clearly. There are deep psychological analyses available in ancient texts of why chanting can help in progressing toward greater freedom and tranquillity, and how the rules are related to this goal.

Sri Krishnamacharya considered Vedic chanting very important, and continued to chant even when he was 100 years of age (to hear Sri Krishnamacharya chanting, please visit www.svastha.com). The branch of the Vedas that he traditionally belonged to is chanted using three notes—*udaata*: the middle note, *anudaata*: one note lower, and *svarita*: one note higher. These rules have been clearly stated in the traditional texts like the *Taittiriya-Praatishaakya*. It is important to make no mistake in this, because when words are juxtaposed or separated in the Vedas, their notes can change, and, to understand how these changes occur, it is essential that the basic notes be understood correctly. This is important not only in chanting, but in meditation as well, because all the Vedic mantras used in meditation also have notes.

Q. What about yoga psychology?

A. Unlike other areas of yoga, there is absolutely no room for confusion in yoga psychology. This is because it depends only on an understanding of the human mind—which has not changed at all since the time of the ancients, and for which we require not advanced technology, but undisturbed tranquillity and awareness.

Consequently, in the area of yoga psychology, there is extensive, clear, and unambiguous information and analysis available in the *Yoga-Sutras*. The *Yoga-Sutras* are exquisitely logical, and the psychology explained in the sutras stands on the strength of its logic alone.

Unfortunately, many well-known, widely recommended contemporary books on the *Yoga-Sutras* and the psychology of yoga are not consistently rational or authentic—they contradict themselves or major commentaries on the *Yoga-Sutras*. We will write further on the *Yoga-Sutras* and yoga psychology in a separate work.

Q. You seem to be against many authors on yoga!

A. No, not at all. I am simply pointing out that contemporary teachers and authors on yoga have the responsibility to present their own ideas as their own. They should not claim to represent the views of a respected and valuable ancient text when in fact their views do not reflect the explanations of the major commentaries on the text, or stand up to rational enquiry. This only does disservice to the many great people in the past who have devoted great selfless effort to explaining the text. Also, these commentaries have been carefully questioned and validated by many other individuals over many centuries, and we stand to gain much by reading and understanding some of these works.

Q. You seem to be critical in your views. Why?

A. I am not being critical, merely factual. Intellectual honesty is an essential quality in a sincere yoga teacher or practitioner. It is better to leave the things that we do not understand alone, rather than act as if we did understand and thereby mislead others and, in the process, stray from the path ourselves. The issues I have raised above have been stated strongly but truly and with reason. You and I will pass away, but the message of the *Yoga-Sutras* is timeless. It delineates a path to freedom from unhappiness, a way to become more complete in yourself. Countless people before us have spent a large portion of their lives exploring and later explaining this path to others. They did this, not because it would be published and they stood to gain materially from it, but because they found the teaching valuable and felt that it was their duty to record it, so that someone at some later time might benefit from it. The integrity and content of this message must not be misrepresented.

About the Authors

THE MOHANS live in India where they have a private yoga therapy practice. They offer comprehensive training programs on yoga and Ayurveda for fitness and therapy under the banner of Svastha Yoga Ayurveda.

Website: www.svastha.com
Email: info@svastha.com

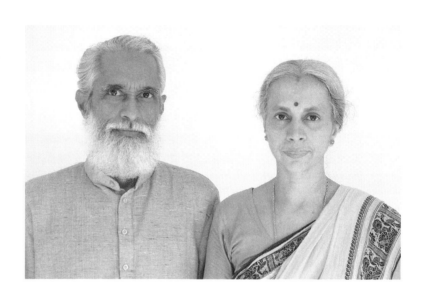

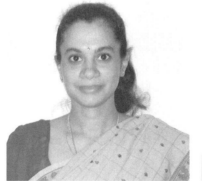
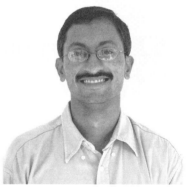